Help! I'm Dying Again

Help! I'm Dying Again

Overcoming Health Anxiety with Cognitive Behavioral Therapy (CBT)

DR BRITNEY CHESWORTH

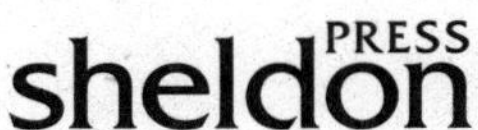

First published by Sheldon Press in 2025
An imprint of John Murray Press

1

A CIP catalogue record for this title is available from the British Library

Trade Paperback ISBN 978 1 399 81582 6
ebook ISBN 978 1 399 81583 3

Typeset by KnowledgeWorks Global Ltd.

Printed and bound in the United States of America.

John Murray Press policy is to use papers that are natural, renewable and recyclable products and made from wood grown in sustainable forests. The logging and manufacturing processes are expected to conform to the environmental regulations of the country of origin.

John Murray Press
Carmelite House
50 Victoria Embankment
London EC4Y 0DZ

www.sheldonpress.co.uk

John Murray Press, part of Hodder & Stoughton Limited
An Hachette UK company

The authorised representative in the EEA is Hachette Ireland,
8 Castlecourt Centre, Dublin 15, D15 XTP3, Ireland (email: info@hbgi.ie)

To my husband, Don, who has endured my many "diagnoses" with endless patience and compassion. Thank you for being my constant when anxiety gets the best of me.

Contents

About the author

Dr. Britney Chesworth is a licensed psychotherapist with a private practice, focusing exclusively on the treatment of anxiety and anxiety-related disorders. She has over 15 years of experience treating clients with anxiety in child welfare, hospice, hospital, university, community mental health and private practice settings. Dr. Chesworth teaches graduate and undergraduate students and mental health professionals on the use of cognitive behavioral therapy (CBT), exposure therapy and other evidence-based interventions. Dr. Chesworth is passionate about using CBT to help others overcome anxiety, as she has personally struggled with it for most of her life.

In addition to her work as a psychotherapist, Dr. Chesworth is a mental health influencer and expert author for *Psychology Today*. She grew up in California and currently resides in Los Angeles with her husband and two children.

Letter to the reader

Dearest health-anxious companions,

Health anxiety is brutal. Believe me, I know. I've spent my fair share of time crippled by irrational fears: heights, enclosed spaces, cats, dogs, spiders, disease, death, what people think, medication, flying, the future, the past, the symptoms of anxiety itself.

Although all of it has sucked in its own unique way, nothing has ravaged me like the fear of disease and death. Still, my story doesn't stop there. Although I do know what it is like to be consumed by these fears, I also know what it is like to feel better. Cognitive behavioral therapy helped me. It has helped the many health-anxious clients I've worked with in my private practice. And it can help you.

In this book, I share stories about all the lumps, moles, aches and pains that have sent me and my clients into a tailspin of problematic thoughts, beliefs and behaviors. I use these stories to teach you strategies to develop healthier thoughts, beliefs and behaviors and overall to help you begin to see health and disease from a fresh, adaptive perspective.

Whether you are in great health, managing a serious illness or somewhere in between, I hope this book helps you feel more understood, empowered and optimistic. You aren't alone. And it can get better. It involves making small but intentional and consistent changes in your thoughts and behaviors each day.

Britney

1

Introduction

When I am chatting with someone about the work I do in my private practice and I use the term *health anxiety*, this is sometimes met with a puzzled expression or a few follow-up questions about what health anxiety is, exactly. This term is becoming increasingly recognized but is not as well-known as other terms that have been more widely used to describe this phenomenon, such as hypochondria. I think it will be useful to briefly break down the meaning of various terms so we can move forward with a common consensus of the key concepts discussed throughout this book.

DSM diagnoses related to health anxiety

Health anxiety is the excessive fear of having or eventually developing a serious disease. Hypochondriasis is the mental disorder that often comes to mind when people think of one experiencing severe anxiety about their health. This was the classification in an older version of the *Diagnostic and Statistical Manual of Mental Disorders* (or the DSM-IV). However, medical and mental health professionals have stopped using the term 'hypochondriac,' as it is outdated and further alienates people experiencing this type of anxiety, many of whom already feel alone, invalidated and misunderstood.

Many people with health anxiety do, indeed, have very real symptoms that are distressing. These symptoms may be part of a medical condition or may be medically unexplained. To diagnose a patient with hypochondriasis, doctors first had to rule out a medical condition. This meant patients experiencing health anxiety *and* real physical symptoms and conditions could not receive this diagnosis. This rigid classification also perpetuated the false assumption of mind–body dualism (i.e. the belief that mind and body are entirely separate entities when they are inherently and inextricably interconnected) and the idea that any medically unexplained symptoms are psychogenic or 'all in your head.'

In response to criticism about the definition and classification of hypochondriasis, it was replaced in the DSM-5 with two new diagnoses:[1]

- Illness Anxiety Disorder (IAD)
- Somatic Symptom Disorder (SSD)

Both of these diagnoses involve the excessive fear of disease, but SSD requires the presence of one or more (often many) somatic symptoms (ranging from moderate to severe), whereas IAD usually involves no symptoms or very mild symptoms. Whether or not you have physical symptoms and/or a medical diagnosis, to meet the criteria for SSD or IAD your anxiety must be excessive and disproportionate to the seriousness of the illness or threat of illness. According to the DSM-5, 75 percent of patients who would have met the criteria for the former hypochondriasis diagnosis now meet the criteria for SSD.[2] However, this estimate has been challenged by research conducted since the release of the DSM-5 and, overall, there are not enough studies to support this assertion.[3]

Defining 'health anxiety'

The information provided up to this point is aimed to offer a 'big picture' of health anxiety and its associated diagnoses. However, you do not need to determine your own classification to benefit from this book, as that is the job of your therapist or other healthcare provider. Health anxiety can be conceptualized as a continuum, with DSM diagnoses (i.e. IAD, SSD) being on the extreme end of that continuum.[3]

For simplicity, the term 'health anxiety' will be used here as the broad, umbrella term to describe 'the experience of excessive fear of disease or preoccupation about one's health,' regardless of whether or not the anxiety is accompanied by a medical condition or meets the criteria for any mental disorder. If you bought this book, you likely identify with this umbrella term and, if so, it is my goal that the strategies taught in this book will help to improve your health anxiety.

When concerns about health become maladaptive

Anxiety is adaptive in particular situations and in moderate doses.[4] If you are in legitimate danger, such as being chased by someone who intends to harm you, then the adaptive, physiological response (i.e. the fight-or-flight response) may be the very thing that keeps you alive. For example, the spike in adrenaline can give you a renewed sense of energy and alertness that helps you escape. Further, even when you are not in danger, small doses of anxiety can serve a positive purpose. If you have an important upcoming exam, a little bit of anxiety can motivate you to study so that you are adequately prepared. However, anxiety becomes a problem in high doses and when it takes over your life.

Similarly, being aware of changes in our bodies and being responsive to potential health threats is adaptive and necessary. However, it becomes maladaptive when the fear of disease or dying becomes so insurmountable that our attempts to ensure health and safety take over our life. So, what does health anxiety look like in our day-to-day lives? It manifests differently in all of us, but there are a few common core features that can help you discern whether your concern over your health has become maladaptive.

The key term to keep in mind when evaluating your experience with health anxiety is *excess*. In other words, the thoughts, feelings and behavior are excessive and considered disproportionate to the actual threat of illness or the seriousness of the symptoms. For those of you with a medical condition, your fears and reactions to symptoms are likely excessive and impair your ability to function in a normal and adaptive manner. Regardless of your personal circumstances, if you have health anxiety, you likely have noticed its presence in your life just based on how much it can ruin your day.

Notably, there are two subtypes under the DSM-5 IAD diagnosis: *care-seeking* and *care-avoidant*. Some research has suggested that while some engage in either care-seeking or care-avoidant behaviors, many fluctuate between these two types of behavior.[5]

Table 1 Common features of health anxiety

Excessive worry over health
Selective attention to bodily changes, functions or sensations and symptoms
Excessively checking body for symptoms
Regularly seeking reassurance from loved ones
Information-seeking on the internet
Avoidance of all health/disease- or death-related stimuli
Frequent medical consultations
Avoidance of doctors or medical consultations
Excessive and overwhelming fear of having an untreatable/serious disease
Excessive and overwhelming fear of a current medical condition
Overall, fears about health are disproportionate to the reality of the situation and/or make it difficult to function well in life

Throughout this book you will see many different examples of what it can look like to live with health anxiety, including my own experiences as well as those of my clients. Health anxiety can play out in unique ways, depending on many factors, such as the person's specific beliefs, fears, thoughts, emotional reactions, symptoms and behaviors. In Chapter 1, I provide a very detailed breakdown of the cycle of health anxiety, including how core beliefs, thoughts and reactions can make daily life rather difficult.

Comorbidities

Health anxiety, regardless of whether it is debilitating enough to meet the criteria for an IAD or SSD diagnosis, is often present alongside other mental health diagnoses. When more than one medical or mental health diagnosis is present, it is referred to as a 'comorbidity' in the healthcare profession. Health anxiety has a particularly high comorbidity rate with panic disorder (PD), obsessive compulsive disorder (OCD) and generalized anxiety disorder (GAD).[3,6,7,8,9]

The strong link between these disorders is not surprising, as characteristics of health anxiety can be seen in core features of each of these disorders: the hyper focus on bodily sensations that occurs with PD; the obsessive thoughts about illness and compulsive rituals or safety behaviors seen in OCD; and the excessive worry that is a salient feature of GAD.[3,6,7,8,9] OCD may be a comorbid diagnosis with IAD or SSD or someone may experience health anxiety as a part of their OCD presentation.[8,10] Other conditions that are comorbid with health anxiety are depressive disorders, bipolar disorder, post-traumatic stress disorder (PTSD), some personality disorders, psychosis, other somatic symptom disorders as well as general medical conditions.[3,11,12,13,14]

Having health anxiety can be a trigger for these other mental health issues. Conversely, having another mental health issue or being diagnosed with a medical condition can make you more susceptible to developing health anxiety. Regardless of which came first, managing more than one at the same time can be especially difficult. It is important to address all the challenges that stem from any mental health or medical conditions you struggle with.

Risk factors of health anxiety

The human experience is complicated. All of the ways we differ from one another are influenced by a complex interplay of factors. For example, intelligence is influenced by the home environment and parental involvement as a child, the availability of learning resources, the quality of education, nutrition, sleep, environment enrichment and genetics. Similarly, a combination of social, psychological and biological factors likely played a role in the development of any health anxiety you may have.

Specifically, certain life experiences have been shown to increase susceptibility to developing health anxiety. Personal experience with a serious illness or witnessing a loved one's illness, disability and/or death, or observing a parent struggle with health anxiety while growing up can be risk factors for health anxiety.[11,15,16,17,18] Further, experiencing trauma as a child (e.g. exposure to violence, childhood abuse or neglect) or as an adult can make one more prone to develop health anxiety.[15,17,19] In addition, some studies suggest that facing considerable stress or being exposed to health-threatening information in the media, on social media or in your social circles can increase one's vulnerability to develop health anxiety.[20]

In addition to social or cultural factors, certain psychological factors have been linked to health anxiety. Some research suggests that adults with an insecure attachment style, emotional instability and distress intolerance are most likely to suffer from health anxiety.[15,16,17,21] Further, personality traits, such as neuroticism or being prone to anxiety, depression and emotional volatility as well as having another psychiatric disorder increases one's likelihood of developing health anxiety.[3,21,22] In addition to all of this, biological factors, such as genetic inheritability of health anxiety, can play a role in its development.[23]

Health anxiety is complicated and we don't always know why it begins. For some it might be obvious. Perhaps a few factors primed the individual, making them vulnerable, and then one triggering event took place (e.g. the death of a loved one, getting a medical diagnosis, entering medical school), in which they suddenly became aware of new fears related to their health. For others, however, there might not have been a clear starting point or pathway but as time went by, they noticed an increasing hypervigilance about health-related matters.

No matter how it starts, once health anxiety develops, it takes on a life of its own. The individual begins to engage in dysfunctional thoughts, beliefs and behaviors that feed the anxiety. They enter a vicious cycle that strengthens over time and becomes increasingly difficult to break free from. For this reason, when it comes to improving health anxiety, the most important question is not about *why* health anxiety developed; if you want to start making changes, the most relevant question is: How is your health anxiety *maintained*?

How health anxiety is maintained

People with health anxiety are not all the same. Each person has their own unique life circumstances, fears, triggers, thoughts and behaviors. However, research suggests common trends among people with health anxiety. Specifically, people with health anxiety tend to hold dysfunctional core beliefs about health and illness (e.g. I am more likely than not to get a serious/terminal illness).

Core beliefs are deeply held beliefs that develop from our significant life experiences; they are the lens through which we interpret what happens in our day-to-day lives. Once a belief develops, we continually reinforce it because we inadvertently search for information to support the belief, making it stronger over time (e.g. seeking content in the news and social media on young people getting terminal illnesses).

When we hold problematic core beliefs about health, we interpret events and bodily sensations in a biased way, which are known as 'cognitive distortions' or 'thinking errors'. People with health anxiety engage in more biased interpretations of symptoms and health-related situations than those without health anxiety.[24] These distorted beliefs and thinking patterns increase anxiety, leading one to engage in dysfunctional behaviors in order to feel safe again (e.g. excessively checking their body, seeking reassurance about symptoms, avoidance). All of this is part of the vicious cycle which increases health anxiety over time. We will discuss all of this in greater detail in Chapter 2.

Health anxiety, meet cognitive behavioral therapy

In CBT, one learns how to reshape these problematic thoughts, beliefs and behaviors into those that are more adaptive. CBT is a psychological intervention that is structured, action-oriented, collaborative, educational and skill-based. It is grounded in the 'cognitive model' or the assumption that thoughts and beliefs influence how people feel and behave.[25] In the context of health anxiety, CBT employs a variety of cognitive and behavioral interventions to help you see health and illness in more adaptive, balanced ways. In this book, you will learn a variety of CBT strategies to help you feel less anxious about your health and improve your overall quality of life.

One of the first steps in CBT is to help you better understand the cycle of health anxiety and how the thoughts and behaviors you think are helping you are actually making your life harder. You will subsequently develop skills to help you:

- Build awareness of your cycle of health anxiety through tracking your thoughts and behaviors in a thought record.
- Critically evaluate and identify the thinking errors that tend to be present with health anxiety.
- Use Socratic dialogue and behavioral experiments to help you change problematic thought patterns.
- Replace dysfunctional behaviors with more adaptive behaviors through exposure and response prevention.
- Modify common problematic core beliefs about health and illness.

Ultimately, I want you to build a set of skills that you can use throughout your lifetime. Below is a list of some of the strategies you will learn in this book.

CBT is considered the first-line treatment for health anxiety, given the large body of research supporting its effectiveness. Results from

Table 2 CBT strategies to improve health anxiety

Exploring core values and setting goals
Psycho-education on the cognitive model and cycle of health anxiety
Monitoring, evaluating and analyzing thought and behavior patterns
Reshaping thought patterns through cognitive restructuring exercises
Reshaping behavioral patterns through exposure exercises/fear hierarchies
Using mindfulness exercises to improve attention skills and stay present-focused

multiple meta-analyses determine that CBT for health anxiety is an effective treatment, having a significant and lasting impact on core symptoms related to health anxiety as well as reducing generalized anxiety, depression and physical symptoms.[26,27,28,29] CBT has become increasingly popular, which, unfortunately, has given rise to a few misconceptions. We've discussed what CBT *is*: its basic tenets and key interventions. Now, let's briefly discuss what CBT *isn't*.

Table 3 What CBT is and is not

What CBT is not	What CBT is
CBT is a rigid, one-size-fits-all approach.	CBT uses different protocols to treat different diagnoses. With health anxiety, the focus is on reducing problematic core beliefs related to health, common thinking errors about symptoms and health-related situations as well as reducing the use of safety behaviors and avoidance when one is anxious about their health. However, all these interventions look very different for each person because their specific fears, thoughts, beliefs and behaviors are unique.
CBT teaches you to ignore symptoms.	Your symptoms are not 'all in your head.' Sometimes your symptoms stem from real concerns, whether due to a diagnosed medical condition or symptoms that are medically unexplained. In other cases, the anxiety itself can produce very real symptoms. CBT helps people learn to see symptoms and bodily changes in more adaptive ways while also recognizing the important role of medicine in promoting health.
CBT only teaches positive thinking.	CBT is less about positive thinking and more about *logical* thinking. The goal is to see the situation as realistically as possible. Sometimes our thoughts related to symptoms and health are inaccurate; CBT challenges such thoughts. Other times, however, our thoughts are valid, and we must face difficult realities. In these cases, CBT shifts the focus towards problem-solving, coping, and acceptance.
CBT 'gaslights' you about health concerns.	Collaboration is key. You are the expert on your own thoughts, beliefs and behaviors, and you bring this expertise to the table. Given that the CBT therapist also knows the common patterns of health-anxious people, CBT collaboratively helps you reframe health-related concerns when this is appropriate. Sometimes your concerns are valid, and it is then recognized that necessary medical consultation is an important part of taking care of yourself.

CBT ignores the past.	CBT is a present-focused treatment, but that doesn't mean it only focuses on the present. Typically, in CBT the therapist starts by focusing on the present problems to address the thoughts, beliefs and behaviors that maintain health anxiety as well as initiating ways to teach fundamental cognitive restructuring skills. The past is explored during other phases, such as when restructuring core beliefs, to help one understand how these beliefs developed.
CBT dismisses emotions.	Emotions give us valuable information about what we think and how we behave. In CBT, we focus on changing thoughts to improve emotional states. We also emphasize the importance of learning to accept unpleasant emotions, like anxiety, as a part of being human and as non-threatening. We want to improve one's ability to tolerate distress.

Health anxiety: friend or foe?

All of our behavior is motivated by something. In other words, we believe that there are advantages to doing the things we do or we wouldn't do them. Even if you don't realize it yet, a part of you likely believes there is at least *some* benefit in worrying about your health. It can be useful to examine these assumptions and evaluate their validity. We can start by breaking it down into a list of benefits and costs. I will list a few of the reasons that both my clients and I believed our health anxiety was helping us as well as reasons we believed it was hurting us.

Perceived *benefits* to having health anxiety:

- My health anxiety keeps me more 'in tune' with my body and keeps me aware of any changes, which will allow me to catch a disease in the early stages.
- My health anxiety allows me to be healthier because I am always thinking about my health and going to the doctor to make sure I am okay.
- Sometimes my health anxiety allows me to be more grateful for my health, such as when I get the results of a test back and am relieved to learn everything is clear.

Perceived *costs* to having health anxiety:

- My health anxiety often consumes me and takes over my life, making it difficult to enjoy anything.
- My health anxiety is driving my family and friends crazy, and negatively impacts these relationships.
- During some periods of my life, I spend way too much money and time going to doctors, urgent care and even the ER.
- During other periods of my life, I get so anxious I avoid the doctor.
- I am often too overwhelmed to concentrate at work, and I take sick days when it becomes too much.
- Living in a continual state of fear has given me a lot of weird anxiety symptoms, which only stresses me out even more.
- All of this has made me more depressed and I don't enjoy things the way I used to.

In exploring the costs and benefits of health anxiety, we often discover that some of the perceived benefits aren't quite as advantageous as we assumed. For example, although it can seem that those of us with health anxiety are simply more 'in tune' with our body, research suggests that this is actually not the case. In fact, we are more likely to make mistakes in our assessments of bodily changes and sensations.[24] My clients often realize this when they reflect on how often they have been wrong about a symptom versus the minimal number of times they have been right.

When my clients reconsider their assumption that their health anxiety keeps them healthy, they often realize that, in all or most cases, obsessing about their bodies or going to the doctor frequently hasn't actually prevented a disease and, instead, has only made life harder unnecessarily. Some research suggests that those with health anxiety are actually *less* likely to engage in health-promoting behaviors than those without health anxiety.[30,31]

As for gratitude, my clients often realize that the relief they feel usually fades quickly and the anxiety often returns. This is consistent with the research underscoring the short-term relief of using problematic behaviors to cope with health anxiety, such as seeking reassurance from doctors and tests.

In later chapters, you will learn how to conduct a detailed cost–benefit analysis to evaluate the benefits and costs of your specific beliefs and behaviors. As a first step, I want you to consider all of the costs and benefits of living with health anxiety. When you are done, remember to reconsider your benefits and reframe any misconceptions or inaccurate assumptions. This exercise can help motivate you to put in the necessary time and effort to complete the other exercises in this book and make some changes about how you deal with your health anxiety.

Envisioning how life could be different

Now that you have evaluated how your health anxiety impacts your life, consider how you would like your life to look different. Having this picture in mind can help you set specific, realistic goals that you would like to work toward while reading this book. Imagine that you wake up tomorrow and, magically, all of your health anxiety is gone. How does your life look different? My client Dan was able to picture a lot of positive changes.

- My wife and I would joke more again and talk about the things we have in common rather than spending so much time talking about my symptoms and fears.
- My friends and I would get together again more.
- My best friend wouldn't get frustrated with me about my constant worrying and bringing up my health concerns.
- I would have time to enjoy surfing, traveling and reading again.
- I would enjoy being an engineer again and would feel good about myself at work.
- I would have more energy to go to the gym and do circuit training three times a week.
- I wouldn't be bogged down by continual fear and looking for signs of disease.
- I would sleep better.
- I would think more clearly.
- I would be in a better mood.
- I could use the money I spend on unnecessary medical expenses for other things—fixing things around the house, weightlifting again.

I encourage you to try this exercise. It can be helpful to consider this in light of your core values or what is most important to you in life.

Some examples of core values include relationships, work, home life, spirituality, religion, interests and hobbies, physical health, mental health, finances and passion projects. Spend a few minutes reflecting on and writing down the daily details of how you would feel, think and behave without the daily burden of health anxiety. How could improving health anxiety change your life, based on the core values that are most important to you?

A few questions to consider during this exercise:

- How would your relationships change or improve? Would this change be noticed by your children, partner, friends, relatives? What would look different in your daily interactions with loved ones?
- Would you notice a difference in your career? How would this affect your relationships with colleagues, interest in work, productivity and satisfaction?
- How would it impact you physically (e.g. energy levels, physical symptoms, nutrition, exercise, sleep)? How has health anxiety taken a toll on you physically?
- Are there activities you would spend more time doing? What hobbies have you put to the side because of health anxiety?
- Are there opportunities you might take advantage of? Is there anything you have missed out on because of health anxiety?
- Would this change make a difference in your finances? What have you spent money on to address your health anxiety?
- How would your life at home look different? Is there anything related to the management of your home life with your family or your responsibilities?

Getting the most out of this book

My hope is that the concepts and exercises in this book help you to interrupt the vicious cycle of health anxiety. I have a few recommendations to help you maximize the value of what you will learn.

As a first step, it can be helpful to know the 'big picture' of how CBT will help you reduce your anxiety. In Chapter 2, you will learn all about the cycle of problematic thoughts, beliefs and behaviors that are keeping your health anxiety alive and well. Building this awareness is an important step to complete prior to making changes.

Each of the subsequent chapters is dedicated to helping you modify key dysfunctional beliefs associated with health anxiety. To reinforce this 'big picture', I recommend you skim through the table of contents and each of the chapters prior to diving into the work in this book.

Secondly, *pace yourself* while working through this book. I recommend reading no more than one chapter per week. Each chapter contains exercises that are critical for solidifying your learning as well as guiding you through the process of changing your thoughts, beliefs and behaviors. I always tell my clients that simply coming to therapy one hour per week is not enough to make a lasting impact on their anxiety. They must dedicate a little bit of time each day to the exercises. Similarly, if you simply read through this book without using the exercises to change your outlook and practice new skills, you will hinder learning and skill acquisition. Thus, it will be important to give yourself time throughout the week to complete the exercises in each chapter.

Thirdly, *work through the chapters in order.* In CBT, we teach certain skills first in order to benefit from those skills while learning subsequent skills. For example, it is important for you to learn how to challenge problematic thoughts (i.e. develop cognitive restructuring skills) prior to engaging in behavioral tasks, such as exposures and experiments. This is because behavioral tasks can sometimes be intimidating and, thus, you will be more likely to succeed in completing them if you know how to effectively challenge problematic thoughts that may arise during these tasks. The chapters in this book are structured so that you build skills in the appropriate, sequential manner.

Lastly, *try not to be hard on yourself* while working through this book. Remember that it likely took you years to strengthen your unhelpful beliefs and become dependent on problematic behaviors. It will take time to change all of this too and that is okay. You will still have good and bad days, weeks, months. Change is not always linear. Give yourself some grace when you find yourself slipping into thinking and behavior that aren't helpful. At the same time, hold yourself accountable to continue putting in the work. You can improve your health anxiety over time through making small, intentional and consistent changes in your thoughts and behaviors each day.

References

1 Bailer J, Kerstner T, Witthöft M, Diener C, Mier D, Rist F. Health anxiety and hypochondriasis in the light of DSM-5. *Anxiety, Stress, & Coping*. 2016;29(2):219–39.

2 American Psychiatric Association. Diagnostic and Statistical Manual of Mental Disorders (DSM-5-TR). Psychiatry.org. Published 2013. <https://www.psychiatry.org/psychiatrists/practice/dsm>

3 Kikas K, Werner-Seidler A, Upton E, Newby J. Illness Anxiety disorder: A review of the current research and future directions. *Curr Psychiatry Rep*. 2024 Jul;26(7):331–339. doi: 10.1007/s11920-024-01507-2. Epub 2024 May 15. PMID: 38748190; PMCID: PMC11211185.

4 Morris DW. Adaptive Affect: The nature of anxiety and depression. *Neuropsychiatric Disease and Treatment*. 2019;15:3323–3326. <https://doi.org/10.2147/ndt.s230491>

5 Newby JM, Hobbs MJ, Mahoney AEJ, Wong S (Kelvin), Andrews G. DSM-5 illness anxiety disorder and somatic symptom disorder: Comorbidity, correlates, and overlap with DSM-IV hypochondriasis. *Journal of Psychosomatic Research*. 2017;101(1):31–37. <https://doi.org/10.1016/j.jpsychores.2017.07.010>

6 Weck F, Bleichhardt G, Witthöft M, Hiller W. Explicit and implicit anxiety: Differences between patients with hypochondriasis, patients with anxiety disorders, and healthy controls. *Cognitive Therapy and Research*. 2010;35(4):317–325. <https://doi.org/10.1007/s10608-010-9303-5>

7 Olatunji BO, Deacon BJ, Abramowitz JS. Is hypochondriasis an anxiety disorder? *British Journal of Psychiatry*. 2009;194(6):481–482. <https://doi.org/10.1192/bjp.bp.108.061085>

8 Hedman E, Ljótsson B, Axelsson E, Andersson G, Rück C, Andersson E. Health anxiety in obsessive compulsive disorder and obsessive compulsive symptoms in severe health anxiety: An investigation of symptom profiles. *Journal of Anxiety Disorders*. 2017;45:80–86. <https://doi.org/10.1016/j.janxdis.2016.11.007>

9 Abramowitz JS, Olatunji BO, Deacon BJ. Health anxiety, hypochondriasis, and the anxiety disorders. *Behavior Therapy*. 2007;38(1):86–94. <https://doi.org/10.1016/j.beth.2006.05.001>

10 Rachman S. Health anxiety disorders: A cognitive construal. *Behaviour Research and Therapy*. 2012;50(7–8):502–512. <https://doi.org/10.1016/j.brat.2012.05.001>

11 Pandey S, Parikh MN, Brahmbhatt MJ, Vankar GK. Clinical study of illness anxiety disorder in medical outpatients. *Archives of Psychiatry and Psychotherapy*. 2017;19(4):32–41. doi:10.12740/APP/76932.

12 Scarella TM, Laferton JAC, Ahern DK, Fallon BA, Barsky A. The relationship of hypochondriasis to anxiety, depressive, and somatoform disorders. *Psychosomatics*. 2016;57(2):200–207.<https://doi.org/10.1016/j.psym.2015.10.006>

13 Pan B, Zhang Q, Tsai H, Zhang B, Wang W. Hypochondriac concerns and correlates of personality styles and affective states in bipolar I and II disorders. *BMC Psychiatry*. 2018;18(1). <https://doi.org/10.1186/s12888-018-1988-0>

14 Lebel S, Mutsaers B, Tomei C, et al. Health anxiety and illness-related fears across diverse chronic illnesses: A systematic review on conceptualization, measurement, prevalence, course, and correlates. Kavushansky A, ed. *PLOS ONE*. 2020;15(7). <https://doi.org/10.1371/journal.pone.0234124>

15 Reiser SJ, Power HA, Wright KD. Examining the relationships between childhood abuse history, attachment, and health anxiety. *Journal of Health Psychology*. 2019;26(7):1085–1095. <https://doi.org/10.1177/1359105319869804>

16 Alberts NM, Hadjistavropoulos HD. Parental illness, attachment dimensions, and health beliefs: Testing the cognitive-behavioural and interpersonal models of health anxiety. *Anxiety, Stress, & Coping*. 2013;27(2):216–228. <https://doi.org/10.1080/10615806.2013.835401>

17 Le TL, Geist R, Bears E, Maunder RG. Childhood adversity and attachment anxiety predict adult symptom severity and health anxiety. *Child Abuse & Neglect*. 2021;120:105216. <https://doi.org/10.1016/j.chiabu.2021.105216>

18 Wright KD, Reiser SJ, Delparte CA. The relationship between childhood health anxiety, parent health anxiety, and associated constructs. *Journal of Health Psychology*. 2015;22(5):617–626. <https://doi.org/10.1177/1359105315610669>

19 Reiser SJ, McMillan KA, Wright KD, Asmundson GJG. Adverse childhood experiences and health anxiety in adulthood. *Child Abuse & Neglect*. 2014;38(3):407–413. <https://doi.org/10.1016/j.chiabu.2013.08.007>

20 McMullan RD, Berle D, Arnáez S, Starcevic V. The relationships between health anxiety, online health information seeking, and cyberchondria: Systematic review and meta-analysis. *Journal of Affective Disorders*. 2019;245:270–278. <https://doi.org/10.1016/j.jad.2018.11.037>

21 Sherry DL, Sherry SB, Vincent NA, et al. Anxious attachment and emotional instability interact to predict health anxiety: An extension of the interpersonal model of health anxiety. *Personality and Individual Differences*. 2014;56:89–94. <https://doi.org/10.1016/j.paid.2013.08.025>

22 Nikčević AV, Marino C, Kolubinski DC, Leach D, Spada MM. Modelling the contribution of the Big Five personality traits, health anxiety, and COVID-19 psychological distress to generalised anxiety and depressive symptoms during the COVID-19 pandemic. *Journal of Affective Disorders*. 2020;279:578–584. <https://doi.org/10.1016/j.jad.2020.10.053>

23 Taylor S, Thordarson DS, Jang KL, Asmundson GJ. Genetic and environmental origins of health anxiety: A twin study. *World Psychiatry*. 2006;5(1):47–50.

24 Du X, Witthöft M, Zhang T, Shi C, Ren Z. Interpretation bias in health anxiety: A systematic review and meta-analysis. *Psychological Medicine*. Published online November 9, 2022:1–12. <https://doi.org/10.1017/s0033291722003427>

25 Chand SP, Kuckel DP, Huecker MR. Cognitive Behavior Therapy (CBT). National Library of Medicine. Published May 23, 2023. <https://www.ncbi.nlm.nih.gov/books/NBK470241/>

26 Olatunji BO, Kauffman BY, Meltzer S, Davis ML, Smits JAJ, Powers MB. Cognitive-behavioral therapy for hypochondriasis/health anxiety: A meta-analysis of treatment outcome and moderators. *Behaviour Research and Therapy*. 2014;58:65–74. <https://doi.org/10.1016/j.brat.2014.05.002>

27 Cooper K, Gregory JD, Walker I, Lambe S, Salkovskis PM. Cognitive behaviour therapy for health anxiety: A systematic review and meta-analysis. *Behavioural and Cognitive Psychotherapy*. 2017;45(2):110–123. <https://doi.org/10.1017/s1352465816000527>

28 Liu J, Gill NS, Teodorczuk A, Li Z, Sun J. The efficacy of cognitive behavioural therapy in somatoform disorders and medically unexplained physical symptoms: A meta-analysis of randomized controlled trials. *Journal of Affective Disorders*. 2019;245:98–112. <https://doi.org/10.1016/j.jad.2018.10.114>

29 Axelsson E, Hedman-Lagerlöf E. Cognitive behavior therapy for health anxiety: Systematic review and meta-analysis of clinical efficacy and health economic outcomes. *Expert Review of Pharmacoeconomics & Outcomes Research*. 2019;19(6):663–676. <https://doi.org/10.1080/14737167.2019.1703182>

30 Fink P, Ørnbøl E, Christensen KS. The outcome of health anxiety in primary care. A two-year follow-up study on health care costs and self-rated health. Baune BT, ed. *PLoS ONE*. 2010;5(3):e9873. <https://doi.org/10.1371/journal.pone.0009873>

31 Yıldız E, Çevik, BE, Güler N. Health anxiety level and health-promoting and protective behaviors of nursing students. *Journal of Education and Research in Nursing*. 2022;19(4):422–428. Accessed November 5, 2024. <https://jer-nursing.org/jvi.aspx?un=JERN-93709&volume=19&issue=4>

2

Understand Health Anxiety

If you are reading this book, you obviously recognize health anxiety as a problem in your life. But that doesn't do you a lot of good if you don't know specifically *how* it is making life harder and *what* to do to change it. If my engine started sputtering and spitting out smoke randomly on my drive to the grocery store, I would know I have a problem. But I would not be able to pop the hood, recognize what's causing the problem and fix it. To improve health anxiety, you need to first understand how your thoughts, beliefs and behaviors are keeping your anxiety alive and well. I would not have been able to make progress with my own health anxiety if I hadn't first learned about how what I thought was helping me was actually *hurting* me.

See, a lot more is happening behind the scenes of health anxiety than you realize. In this chapter, I am going to give you the 'big picture' of the thoughts, beliefs and behaviors that are making you more anxious about your health. This will set you up for the rest of the chapters in this book, in which I will help you to develop and practice a new set of skills that will allow you to think and behave in new ways. As you read through subsequent chapters, it may be helpful to refer back to this chapter as necessary to review this 'big picture' and all of the key contributors to health anxiety.

The power of your thoughts

We don't give our thoughts enough credit. We know they matter to some extent, of course, but we don't necessarily think of them as playing a significant role in our day-to-day experiences. We pay a lot more attention to the situations or events that take place around us and how we *feel* or what we *do* about those situations.

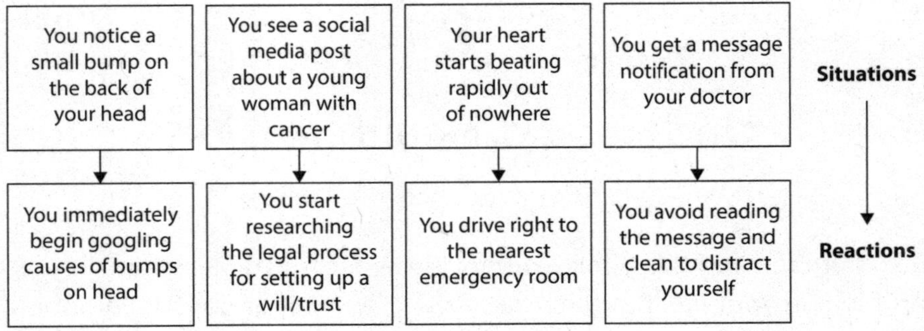
You notice a small bump on the back of your head
You see a social media post about a young woman with cancer
Your heart starts beating rapidly out of nowhere
You get a message notification from your doctor
Situations
You immediately begin googling causes of bumps on head
You start researching the legal process for setting up a will/trust
You drive right to the nearest emergency room
You avoid reading the message and clean to distract yourself
Reactions

So, why do the situations and our reactions get all the attention? It is because we often just assume that a situation happens and then we react directly to that situation. Nope. What is *really* happening is:

- Something happens.
- We *interpret* that situation.
- We react to our interpretation of the situation.

To illustrate, let's look back at the same situations and add in the missing pieces of the puzzle: *our interpretation of the situation.*

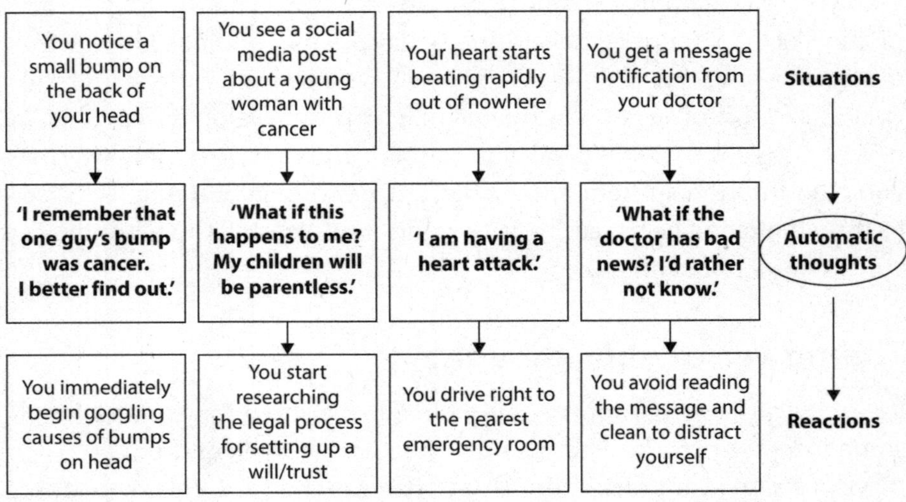
You notice a small bump on the back of your head
You see a social media post about a young woman with cancer
Your heart starts beating rapidly out of nowhere
You get a message notification from your doctor
Situations
'I remember that one guy's bump was cancer. I better find out.'
'What if this happens to me? My children will be parentless.'
'I am having a heart attack.'
'What if the doctor has bad news? I'd rather not know.'
Automatic thoughts
You immediately begin googling causes of bumps on head
You start researching the legal process for setting up a will/trust
You drive right to the nearest emergency room
You avoid reading the message and clean to distract yourself
Reactions

Your emotional and behavioral reactions make a lot more sense when you look at how you interpret situations when it comes to your health. To clarify, a 'situation' could be an event happening in real-time like noticing a new symptom or learning about someone else's health issue. Or it could be something that takes place in your mind, such as a memory of someone you love dying from a disease, or a daydream about you getting a terrible diagnosis. Bearing in mind this definition, a situation happens, you have thoughts about that situation and then you react to those thoughts. It is a simple and obvious concept, yes. But regardless, we tend to neglect this very critical piece: our interpretations or our *automatic thoughts*.

Automatic thoughts are fleeting thoughts that pass through our minds quickly, often without our awareness. They tend not to be deliberate but emerge spontaneously. When we are aware of them, we tend to accept them uncritically. And, friends, this is where the trouble begins! Often, without realizing it, we engage in what are called 'cognitive distortions' or 'thinking errors.' Thinking errors are biased, inaccurate and/or unhelpful thoughts that negatively impact our mood and behavior.

Research shows that people with health anxiety engage in a lot of thinking errors.[1,2] When you interpret health-related situations in a biased way, you experience a lot of unnecessary distress. By identifying any potentially biased thoughts, you give yourself the opportunity to evaluate their validity rather than automatically accept them as valid. Below are several thinking errors commonly experienced by people with health anxiety. I've also included some examples to help illustrate these concepts.

1 Black-and-white thinking (or all-or-nothing thinking)

Viewing health in absolute, black and-white categories instead of taking a more balanced approach and seeing health and illness on a continuum. One is either perfectly healthy or deathly ill.

Examples

Even though the results of my physical were normal and healthy overall, my doctor put me on medication for high blood pressure. Clearly, I am not in good health.
This is the second time this year I have had a bad cough. My health is in ruins.
I couldn't sleep because I am stressed about receiving the test results. If I am diagnosed with diabetes, I might as well start planning my funeral.

2 Jumping to conclusions

Interpreting the meaning of a health-related situation with little or no evidence. This can happen in two ways:

(a) *Fortune telling*: Making negative predictions about what will happen regarding your health when other outcomes are more likely. You predict you will develop a certain type of sickness or you might believe you know exactly what doctors will or will not be able to do to treat a certain health issue.

Examples

Two of my grandparents had dementia so it is inevitable that I will get dementia eventually.
If I ever get diagnosed with cancer, I will probably be screwed. Treatments will probably be useless so I might as well not go through it and embrace my death.

(b) *Mind reading*: Interpreting the thoughts and beliefs of others without adequate evidence. You might make assumptions about what medical professionals or loved ones think about your health.

Examples

My mom had a concerned look on her face when I told her I wasn't feeling well. She thinks it is something serious.
The nurse gave me a look of pity when she called me back to see the doctor. She knows the doctor is getting ready to tell me bad news.

3 Catastrophizing

Predicting only the most disastrous outcomes when it comes to your health. Anytime you have an unexplained bodily sensation or symptom, you find yourself thinking that something is *terribly* wrong.

Examples

My period is irregular this month. It is probably ovarian cancer.
My muscles have been twitching lately. What if it is ALS?
This rash on my leg could be flesh-eating bacteria. It could be too late for me by the time I make it to the doctor.

4 Unrealistic expectations

Expectations that doctors and tests should be able to give you definitive answers or explanations for every potential question, concern or symptom/bodily sensation.

Examples

It is unacceptable that the results of my breast ultrasound state that it is *probably* not cancer. A scan should be able to determine this with 100% certainty.
My neurologist ruled out his concerns with scans and tests. But he wasn't able to tell me why I have been more forgetful lately. How incompetent. Every symptom has an explanation.
The results of this scan only state that there were no abnormalities found. I do not feel at peace with my health like I hoped I would. These results are not very convincing.

5 Mental filter/Tunnel vision

You focus on certain health-related information that supports your health-related beliefs, while ignoring or dismissing the information that challenges your health-related beliefs. You might inundate yourself with tragic stories about illness and death in the news and in your social networks. However, you pay a lot less attention to the many stories about healthy people or those who recover from an illness.

Examples

Someone I knew from college died of a brain aneurysm. She was in her thirties. This is exactly why I am always vigilant about my health. Young people die from serious diseases all of the time.
There are so many stories about young people getting diagnosed with serious health issues. I read and watch videos about it all over social media. Disease is everywhere.
I saw an article about someone with cancer who went through treatment and is now cancer-free. He is one of the lucky few.

6 Emotional reasoning

When you believe that something must be true because it *feels* true, without substantial evidence or when facts support the contrary. This can happen in two ways:
(a) *Anxiety is predictive of health outcomes*: You are convinced that having a strong emotion, such as anxiety, is a sign that something is *terribly* wrong.

Examples

I have a headache today and I never get headaches. Something feels 'off'. This is a premonition that something is seriously wrong with me.
Why am I more anxious than normal about these muscle spasms? This must be a sign that things are not okay.

(b) *The absence of anxiety is predictive of health outcomes*: You are convinced that the absence of anxiety or another unpleasant emotion will inevitably result in a negative health outcome.

Examples

I am not anxious about receiving my test results today. This probably means I am going to be surprised with bad news.
I am getting an ultrasound today and I haven't been thinking about it. But this is what happens. Someone isn't worried about their symptoms and then, when they go in to get their test results, they are hit with shocking news.

7 Overgeneralization

Making a broad negative conclusion about many or all situations based on one or a few health-related events or situations.

Examples

My friend had a hard time getting an accurate diagnosis because her first doctor didn't order the test needed to identify the problem. Doctors are lazy and incompetent.
I know someone who experienced dizziness and fainted. She didn't go to the doctor because she assumed it was due to perimenopause. It ended up being due to a brain tumor. This shows me how important it is to be extra diligent and go to the doctor right away with every new symptom or sensation.
Treatment didn't work for my neighbor. We need to stay away from western medicine.

8 Magical thinking

Assuming thoughts or acts will influence unrelated events (about health).

Examples

I need to stop worrying that I have dementia or I am going to manifest it.
I can't believe that a commercial just came on about breast cancer. I was worried about having breast cancer just last night. This must be a sign from the universe that I have it.
Nope—I will not say the 'c-word' (cancer) or I am going to get it.

In reviewing these thinking errors, I hope you identified those that impact you the most. My clients often tell me that they have engaged in most of these at one point or another, but two or three *really* pop out at them. Remember, your thoughts are powerful! They have a significant impact on the way you feel and the things you do throughout your day. Understanding the common thinking errors and building awareness of your thought patterns is an important step in improving health anxiety.

Internal health anxiety triggers and body vigilance

Distressing thoughts about our health don't come out of nowhere. We are triggered in some way. In the diagrams at the beginning of the chapter, the 'event' or 'situation' is typically the trigger. Triggers can be *internal* or *external*. Internal triggers include intrusive or distressing thoughts or bodily sensations and symptoms. Distressing or intrusive thoughts might be images or thoughts that pop into one's head about getting a disease and suffering or dying.

When it comes to health anxiety, thinking errors are most often triggered by bodily sensations and symptoms. Take a look at the list of bodily sensations. Most people experience these sensations periodically. As you look through this list, consider each one and check off any that have triggered anxiety at some point. Also, consider any additional sensations not listed here.

Table 1 Internal health threat triggers or common symptoms or bodily sensations

• Difficulty swallowing • Body aches, pains or cramps • Heart racing or palpitations • Dizziness or lightheadedness • Twitches • Difficulty breathing • Nausea • Changes in appetite • Bloating • Sores or pimples	• Blurred vision • Sweaty or warm • Weak or tired • Dry mouth • Muscle tension or weakness • Chest discomfort (tightness, pain) • Hot flashes • Chills • Scratchy or sore throat • Heartburn • Fatigue or excessive tiredness • Eye discomfort • Changes in hearing	• Headache • Congestion • Tingling or numbness • Dry mouth • Diarrhea or constipation • Insomnia • Restlessness or on edge • Difficulty concentrating • Skin itchiness or blemishes • Forgetfulness or confusion • Other

People with health anxiety tend to engage in what is called 'body vigilance.'[3,4] Body vigilance is when you closely monitor your body for symptoms and bodily sensations. Health-anxious people tend to be hypervigilant about bodily symptoms and sensations because they mistakenly assume that most or all bodily sensations or symptoms are threatening and due to an underlying disease. In reality, our bodies are 'noisy' and we can have symptoms because of normal self-regulatory biological processes, diet, anxiety and benign or minor medical conditions.

The problem with body vigilance is that it makes you more likely to notice bodily sensations and symptoms. In addition, when you experience anxiety, it can produce even more sensations due to the physiological sensations that accompany anxiety (i.e. the fight-flight-freeze response or mind–body connection). Further, you then try to assess or find the cause for every bodily sensation, which leads you to misinterpret harmless or benign bodily sensations as a sign of a disease. And, *voilà*, you have entered thinking error territory. In a later chapter, we will dive into body vigilance in more depth to help you improve your fear of bodily sensations.

External health anxiety triggers

While internal triggers involve being triggered by something that happens within your body, external triggers include situations or events that take place in the environment or any external stimuli. Like internal triggers, external stimuli can signal a current or future health concern and, therefore, create a lot of anxiety. Some examples are learning about cancer rates, hearing a scary health story or being exposed to someone ill. Take a look at the brief list below and check off any that have triggered your health anxiety.

External health threat triggers:

- Scary health-related topics in the news
- Sad or tragic personal health stories on social media
- Being in contact with sick people because they might be contagious
- Being exposed to germs in public spaces
- Seeing a loved one suffer from an illness or die
- Learning that someone you know has been diagnosed with an illness
- An upcoming medical appointment or test

- Receiving inconclusive or dissatisfactory results of a test
- Being away from familiar healthcare facilities
- Learning that you have a health condition
- Having a difficult or traumatic experience in the healthcare system
- Other

Building thought awareness

One of the first tasks I do with my health-anxious clients is to teach them how to monitor and track their thoughts about their health. Learning how to recognize thoughts and identify potential thinking errors is a skill. As with any skill, the more you practice monitoring your thoughts, the easier it will be to recognize problematic thoughts automatically as you go about your day.

Start by tracking situations and thoughts that took place in the recent past. Think of a time over the past week or two when you felt anxious about your health. Begin with that situation and fill in all of the relevant information. Next, try to document situations and thoughts as they happen throughout the week. Documenting your thoughts doesn't have to be a big commitment. Set aside 5 minutes a day to track your thoughts and identify those that seem problematic. See the examples below for guidance and inspiration.

As a bonus tip, if you have a hard time thinking of a situation, start with the feeling. Think of a time recently when you felt particularly anxious about your health, such as an intensity level of around 6/10 or higher. What happened *just before* you started feeling anxious? For example, did you notice a new symptom, get a message from your doctor, hear a story or read something online?

Thought record

Note: Situation is defined as an internal or external trigger. This could be an internal trigger (e.g. noticing a new symptom or bodily sensation or having a health-related thought/image/daydream/memory) or external trigger (e.g. an upcoming medical appointment, getting a diagnosis or learning something new about your health, learning scary health information in the news or hearing a tragic health story, health news about a loved one or being around a sick loved one).

Date & situation or trigger (internal or external) & level of anxiety (1–10)

August 10

I felt bloated and had to pee multiple times within a short period of time.

Anxiety: 7/10

Automatic thought about the situation & level of concern (1–10)

I once read a story online about a woman who had bloating and frequent urination. It turned out she had ovarian cancer. What if I have ovarian cancer?

Level of concern: 6/10

Potential thinking errors

(1) Catastrophizing: thinking of the worst-case scenario and not considering other benign, more likely explanations for my symptoms (e.g. menstruation, I drank a bit more water today).

(2) Mental Filter/Tunnel vision: hyper focusing on the tragic and rare stories and paying less attention to the many stories about healthy people or about situations when myself or others had symptoms and it ended up not being serious.

Date & situation or trigger (internal or external) & level of anxiety (1–10)

August 14

I was feeling confident about my health after the results of my physical but then noticed my eyes are yellowish and jaundice-looking.

Anxiety: 8/10

Automatic thought about the situation & level of concern (1–10)

Of course, as soon as I feel relaxed and don't have anxiety, I am slapped in the face with a new health concern. Now I have a potential new disease to worry about.

Level of concern: 8/10

Potential thinking errors

All-or-nothing thinking: assuming my health is a light switch—on or off—instead of seeing my health as on a continuum. One minute, I am 100 percent healthy, the next minute I am potentially dying from a serious disease.

Emotional reasoning: assuming the absence of anxiety is predictive of future health concerns when the two are unrelated.

Date & situation or trigger (internal or external) & level of anxiety (1–10)

August 18

I read a story in the news about a woman who was misdiagnosed. Doctors thought her symptoms were due to pancreatitis but it turned out it was pancreatic cancer. She died.

Anxiety: 7/10

Automatic thought about the situation & level of concern (1–10)

This is exactly why I don't trust doctors. It's almost a rare event for them to get it right. I have to take matters into my own hands since they clearly don't know what they are doing.

Level of concern: 9/10

Potential thinking errors

(1) Overgeneralization: making general conclusions about all doctors' competency or all tests' effectiveness based on one situation.

(2) Mental filter/Tunnel vision: hyper focusing on one unfortunate story while paying less attention to many others stories: I know about people who were diagnosed accurately and effectively treated for something.

Now that you have gotten a taste of it, keep up the good work! Remember, just as with developing any new skill, you need to practice monitoring your health-related thoughts and building that thought awareness. Eventually, you won't need to document all of your thoughts because you will have established the habit of noticing thoughts as they come.

Building the habit of thought awareness will allow you to take the next step in the process of improving health anxiety: learning how to challenge thinking errors and reshape problematic thinking patterns when it comes to your health. This skill is called 'cognitive restructuring'. You will have the chance to develop and practice cognitive restructuring skills throughout the remaining chapters in this book.

Dysfunctional core beliefs about health and illness

We discussed thinking errors related to health anxiety first because those are surface-level cognitions that are the most obvious to us. However, more is happening beneath the surface. Thinking errors are merely a symptom of the bigger problem: *core beliefs*. Core beliefs are the deeper-level cognitions that are the driving force behind all of your automatic thoughts. You likely engage in a lot of thinking errors about your health *because* you have dysfunctional core beliefs about health and illness.

So, what are core beliefs, exactly? Core beliefs are deeply ingrained beliefs we hold about ourselves, others, the future and the world. They often originate in childhood through personally significant life experiences. These past experiences could be traumatic but they don't have to be. They could simply be adverse or significant events that took place in our lives that were meaningful in some way.

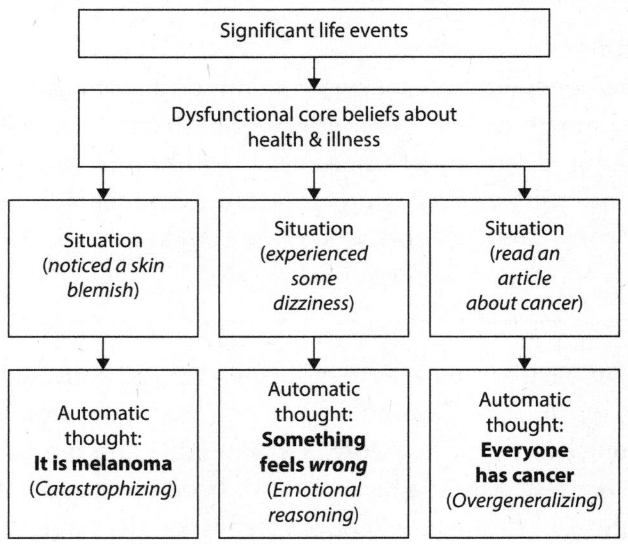

Core beliefs play a powerful role in how we process information. Once they develop and are set in motion, core beliefs are continuously reinforced because we selectively attend to information that confirms our belief and ignore or dismiss information that does not support the belief. In other words, we are on the lookout to find 'evidence' that confirms our beliefs and then we dismiss or ignore any evidence against that belief. This process of reinforcement only makes our beliefs stronger over time.

Researchers have identified several common dysfunctional core beliefs among people with health anxiety.[5,6,7,8] I will briefly list and describe them here but know that we will address each of these beliefs in depth through the remaining chapters of this book.

Table 2 Common core beliefs

Core belief	Description
Overestimate likelihood of a health problem	Belief that diseases are more *common* than they actually are, statistically speaking.
Overestimate severity of a health problem	Belief that diseases are more *severe* than they actually are, statistically speaking.
Intolerance of uncertainty	Belief that one should be able to be 100 percent certain about one's health status at all times or be 100 percent certain that one won't have negative health outcomes.
Vulnerability to sickness & inability to cope	Belief that one is continuously sick or particularly vulnerable to illness and is unable to cope with illness.
Anxiety sensitivity	Belief that the physical sensations associated with anxiety are dangerous and/or that one is unable to tolerate anxiety.
Rigid health beliefs	Belief that, in order to be healthy, one must be 100 percent symptom-free and/or be completely free of any type of health issue (one is either 100 percent sick or 100 percent healthy).
Inadequacy of medical resources	Belief that physicians, medical tests and/or medical treatments are all invalid, ineffective and/or insufficient.
Beliefs about death	Beliefs that death and dying will inevitably be heartbreaking and agonizing experiences to the point that one is unable to cope with or accept it.

How core beliefs develop over time

To help illustrate, let me tell you a little about how my own core beliefs developed and were strengthened over time. Throughout most of my childhood, my mother was in pain. She would get migraines that would last for days and often made her throw up. As a single mother, she had to work but she spent a great deal of her non-work time in bed because the pain was unbearable. Looking back, I don't have very many memories of her without a headache. She rarely complained about it but I knew just by looking at her face. I remember the doctors saying her migraines seemed more severe than most they had encountered but they couldn't figure out what was causing them. Over the years, they ran a number of scans and tests but were unable to identify the source. When I was 16, she died from an overdose of her pain medication.

These experiences with my mother led me to develop certain beliefs about illness at a young age. My health anxiety started around the 5th grade. I began to believe that serious diseases were extremely common and that those who weren't plagued with a debilitating illness were among the lucky few. After all, if my only parent was sick, then so many others out there must be experiencing something similar. I also began to assume that if someone is sick, then it is likely to be very serious and eventually terminal. Even though my mom had some health problems, she had a lot going for her. She was young, took care of herself, had 'good genes', followed her physicians' orders and, yet, she still died. So I concluded that if one is diagnosed with anything, they are as good as dead.

Once these health-related beliefs were solidified, then the process of reinforcement began. Essentially, I would scan my environment and selectively attend to all the pieces of 'evidence' that supported my belief system. I paid special attention to situations when one of our relatives got sick or when I learned that a friend's family member was sick or dying. I read all about various diseases in medical texts. I was overly focused in my 6th grade health class. And I watched as many tragic movies and TV shows about the sick and dying as I could get my hands on. I was so busy seeking out sickness and death that I failed to acknowledge that, aside from my mom, everyone in my life was pretty healthy and, well, alive.

Now, what do you think all of this did to my health-related beliefs? These beliefs just got progressively stronger over the years. How could they not? In the world I had created for myself through all of these activities, everyone was sick and dying! I remember at one point as a teenager, I thought how lucky I was that I had escaped serious disease and death. I laugh at that now. Here I was, a young person with virtually no health issues, and I believed that my survival was some kind of miracle. It demonstrates just how biased and inaccurate my thinking had become through this whole process.

Exploring your own health-related experiences

Your own life experiences that contributed to your health anxiety may not be as obvious or cliché as mine. But I am guessing if you did some digging, you'd find some situations or events that have significantly impacted you. Your health anxiety is likely the culmination of a variety of experiences. It can be helpful initially to understand what triggered the development of inaccurate beliefs. However, as we talked about in the introduction, insight alone isn't enough to improve your health anxiety. It is much more important to understand how your core beliefs are being reinforced in your everyday life and then to make the necessary changes in your thoughts and behaviors to stop that reinforcement process.

Core beliefs are not a permanent state of mind. Anything learned can be unlearned. You can change these beliefs by rewiring or retraining your brain to see yourself and the world around you differently. We will be reshaping core beliefs throughout the rest of the book but, for now, it is important for you to know the process by which these beliefs are maintained as well as their temporary, ever-changing nature.

To help solidify your understanding of these concepts, let's try a brief mental exercise. Review the list of core beliefs above and write down any that resonate. Next, think of any life experiences that may have contributed to the development of this belief. This doesn't need to be an in-depth exercise but just a way for you to start recognizing how core beliefs may have developed in your own life. To help get you started, I added a couple of examples of my own.

Core beliefs	Relevant life experiences
Overestimation of likelihood & severity of health problems	Growing up with a mother who had migraines (and in my mind was 'sick' all the time) made it seem like being very sick was normal and expected (serious disease is common). Also, my mother was only 41 when she died. From this, I concluded that if one is sick, they are likely to die (i.e. all disease is severe or deadly).
Inadequacy of medical resources	Physicians and medical resources/treatments were not able to help my mother. Thus, I concluded that this would be the case for me too. If I were to develop or contract a disease, I might as well start planning my funeral.

Avoidance and safety-seeking behaviors

People with health anxiety tend to use both *avoidance* and *safety-seeking behaviors* as a coping mechanism when they are anxious about their health. Health-anxious people use these coping strategies in an attempt to reduce the anxiety they experience after being triggered by an internal (e.g. a symptom) or external event (e.g. a cancer story). All of these behaviors are used to reach one overarching goal: *to feel safer.* Ironically, however, although these behaviors might reduce anxiety in the moment, they ultimately increase anxiety over the long term. So, what do these behaviors look like? We will discuss avoidance and safety behaviors separately.

Please note that, as discussed in Chapter 1, health-anxious people who meet the criteria for Illness Anxiety Disorder typically fall into one of two categories: the 'care-avoidant' or 'care-seeking' subtype. Thus, as one might expect, care-avoidant subtypes are more likely to use avoidant behaviors and care-seeking subtypes are more likely to use safety behaviors such as reassurance-seeking from the healthcare system.

Avoidance

Avoidance is when a person avoids anything that makes them feel anxious about their health. This can look like skipping physicals or regular check-ups at the doctor or, if they have a concerning symptom, they put off getting it examined by a doctor because they fear being told that something is wrong.

Others with health anxiety avoid anything that reminds them of certain diseases or sickness and death in general. They might not visit people in the hospital, go to funerals or memorials, talk about death, read obituaries, write a will, or engage with media about illness and death. Some health-anxious people avoid anything they believe might lead them to contract an illness, such as going to public or crowded places or visiting ill loved ones.

Lastly, many people with health anxiety avoid any activities that induce physiological sensations or changes in their physiological state because they mistakenly believe that the physiological sensations themselves are dangerous in some way. The most common example I have seen is avoiding exercise of any kind because of fears of an increased heart rate or altered breathing patterns. Some people might also avoid drinking caffeine, eating certain types of foods or having sex.

Safety-seeking behaviors

Safety-seeking behaviors or safety behaviors are what health-anxious people *do* to reduce anxiety and prevent their health fears from coming true. Think of safety behaviors as a subtle form of avoidance in which you put certain safeguards in place to prevent a potential medical crisis or medical disaster. For simplicity, we will break down safety behaviors into three main types: *reassurance-seeking*, *excessive-checking* and *preventive*.

Let's start with *reassurance-seeking behaviors.* To deal with the stress of a new symptom or sensation, you collect information from doctors, other people, or online to assess what kind of danger you might be in. With *excessive-checking behaviors*, you often monitor your own body for symptoms, physical sensations or any kind of bodily function that might be 'concerning.' *Preventive behaviors* are used in an attempt to prevent the possibility of future health problems. A wide variety of behaviors fall under this umbrella. You might keep a strict diet and exercise regimen, or you might have to know where the nearest hospital is at all times.

Avoidance and safety-seeking behaviors increase anxiety

Any time you avoid something, the fear of that thing grows more intense over time. For example, we never give ourselves the chance to learn that we can tolerate going to the doctor or that the changes in our physiological state are not dangerous. Similarly, the more we use safety behaviors, the more meaning and significance we give to them and, thus, the more dependent we become on them to feel safe.

Importantly, it is essential to take reasonable steps to optimized your health. However, safety behaviors are excessive and go beyond what we would consider reasonable steps. We will discuss this in detail in Chapter 6.

Tying it all together to see the 'big picture' of health anxiety

Now that you have learned about the different types of problematic thoughts, beliefs and behaviors, let's take a look at how these components operate together to create an ongoing, vicious cycle of health anxiety. Take a look at the diagram and let's walk through each component of this cycle.

The Vicious Cycle of Health Anxiety

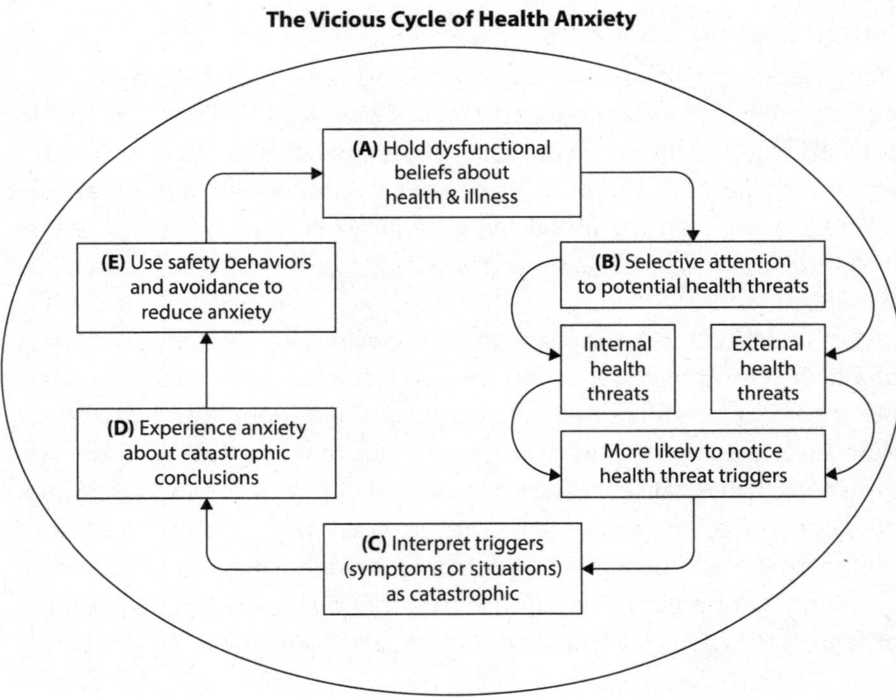

(A) You hold dysfunctional core beliefs about health and illness. These drive the things you think and do on a daily basis.

(B) These beliefs compel you to pay selective attention to health threats. In other words, you actively seek out any information that could point to a current or future health crisis. These 'threats' could be internal or external. In order to identify internal threats or bodily sensations and symptoms, you engage in 'body vigilance' and become hyper aware of any potential noise your body makes (e.g. *'Did my heart just skip a beat? Is that a slight pain in my side?'*). Engaging in body vigilance is the most common way a health-anxious person pays selective attention to health threats. In addition to body vigilance, you might be on the lookout for external health threats, such as scary diseases in the news, tragic health stories on social media or having contact with someone who is sick. Your selective attention to internal and external health threats makes you more likely to notice these triggers.

(C) You then interpret the internal and external triggers in a biased way by engaging in thinking errors. These distorted interpretations lead you to interpret neutral or benign bodily sensations as some sort of catastrophe. For example, you experience a muscle twitch, an internal trigger, and conclude that it is the first sign of multiple sclerosis (MS) (i.e. *catastrophizing thinking error*). Or you hear a tragic health story, an external trigger, and become convinced that people everywhere are dying of cancer so you probably will too (i.e. *overgeneralization thinking error*).

(D) Naturally, your catastrophic conclusions cause anxiety and distress.

(E) You begin to use safety and avoidant behaviors to alleviate your anxiety and prevent a medical crisis (e.g. googling symptoms, repeatedly going to the doctor, excessively checking your body). However, these behaviors don't reduce anxiety or only reduce anxiety temporarily and you never get the opportunity to challenge your dysfunctional beliefs. And then *all of this* only further reinforces your dysfunctional beliefs about health and illness.

So the cycle continues and all of your dysfunctional thoughts, beliefs and behaviors continue to intensify your health anxiety over time.

Erica's cycle of health anxiety

Let's walk through an example of this cycle. My client, Erica, dealt with pretty severe health anxiety.

(A) One of the many inaccurate core beliefs she held was that, in order to be healthy, she had to be symptom-free. She also believed that she was weak or vulnerable and would be unable to cope if she was diagnosed with a disease. These beliefs convinced her that a symptom meant a diagnosis and a diagnosis, in turn, meant impending death. So, naturally, any symptom was a big deal for her.

Erica's Cycle of Health Anxiety

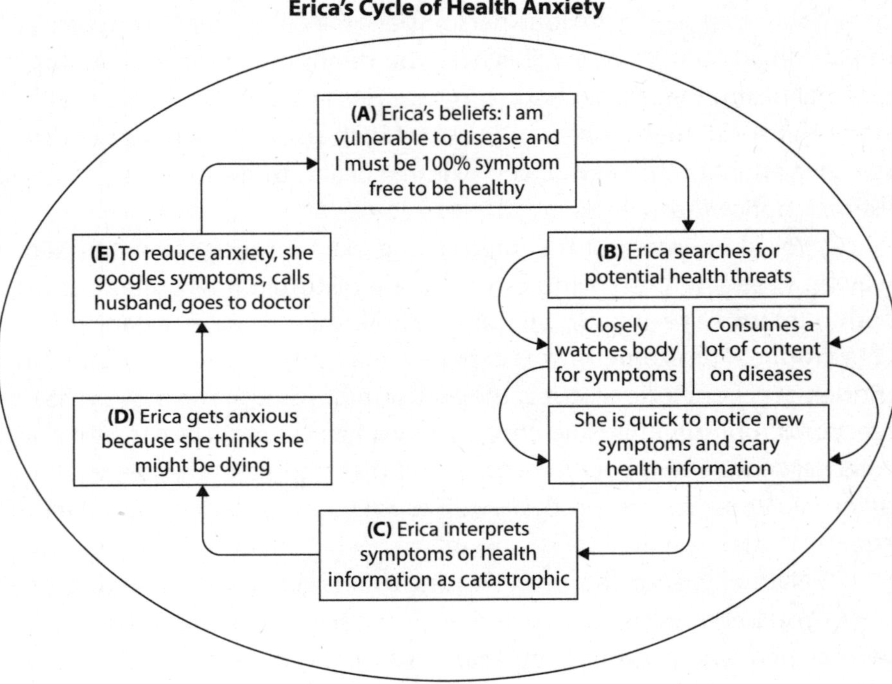

(B) Erica, therefore, engaged in body vigilance and was constantly on the lookout for any new bodily sensations or symptoms. She also sought out information about young people dying from disease on Quora, TikTok and Instagram, news outlets and health websites. Of course, Erica's hyper awareness made her more likely to notice health threats. She was quick to notice new symptoms and seemed to frequently come across troubling information about diseases.

(C) She then interpreted every symptom and situation as a catastrophe. For example, she often diagnosed random bodily sensations as an impending stroke or heart attack.

(D) Erica's catastrophic conclusions understandably led her to experience significant anxiety about her health.

(E) To reduce her anxiety and ensure that she would be okay and not face some sort of a medical crisis, she used safety behaviors. She would call her husband throughout the day to ask if he thought her symptoms were concerning. She spent ample time reading about her symptoms and their various causes on the internet. And she would periodically pop over to her local urgent care when she really thought something was wrong. Erica's safety behaviors sometimes improved her anxiety, at first. But then either the old symptom didn't go away or a new symptom emerged and she was back to square one again.

The cycle continued to repeat itself. By the time Erica came to me for treatment, the time and energy she spent seeking out health threats and engaging in safety behaviors were all-consuming. Her health anxiety had taken over her life.

Identifying your own patterns with health anxiety

This is the overall 'big picture' of health anxiety. Keep in mind that, as with many things in life, health anxiety exists on a spectrum. Your anxiety about your health may not be as bad as Erica's. Or perhaps it is worse. Wherever you land on the spectrum, it is likely that you engage in at least some of these problematic thoughts, beliefs and behaviors. An important step in getting better is to identify your own patterns. This awareness will then pave the way for you to work on changing problematic thoughts and beliefs and reducing your use of unhelpful behaviors. I will help you make these changes throughout the rest of this book.

As a final step in this chapter, let's help you use what you have learned to build awareness of your own patterns. Over the next few days, continue documenting the situations and thoughts as you did earlier in this chapter. However, now I want you to document what you did in response to your health-related concerns as well as identify any potential underlying core beliefs that might be present. At this point, we aren't making judgments about anything, nor are we trying to make any changes in your thoughts or behavior. We are simply observing in order to help you become familiar with your patterns.

Thought record

Note: Situation is defined as an internal or external trigger. This could be an internal trigger (e.g. noticing a new symptom or bodily sensation or having a health-related thought/image/daydream/memory) or external trigger (e.g. an upcoming medical appointment, getting a diagnosis or learning something new about your health, learning scary health information in the news or hearing a tragic health story, health news about a loved one or being around a sick loved one).

Date & situation or trigger & anxiety level (0–10)

August 20

I saw a TikTok video on a woman with three children who was diagnosed with MS.

Anxiety: 6/10

Automatic thought about the situation & level of concern (0–10)

This is why I shouldn't allow myself to feel safe. Young people get diagnosed with serious illnesses all the time. Plus she had kids. What if my kids are left motherless? They will not survive without me.

Level of concern: 6/10

Potential thinking errors

(1) Mental filter/Tunnel vision: hyper focusing on the tragic stories.

(2) Catastrophizing: thinking of the worst-case scenarios—not only will I get a serious illness but I will die from it and my kids will not survive without me.

Actions taken or not taken (safety behaviors & avoidance)

Reassurance seeking: I inadvertently ended up spending hours reading online about MS and other neurological diseases, including symptoms, prognosis and treatment options.

Potential underlying core beliefs behind health concerns

(1) Overestimating likelihood/severity of health problems: assuming serious disease is more common than it is. Also, assuming serious disease is more severe than it likely is. I am assuming I will die while my kids are young instead of recognizing that many people can still live long lives with diseases like MS.

(2) Beliefs about death: death is terrifying to me because I assume that if I die, my children will not survive it.

Date & situation or trigger & anxiety level (0–10)

August 25

Noticed a sharp pain in my breast.

Anxiety: 8.5/10

Automatic thought about the situation & level of concern (0–10)

What if I have breast cancer like my aunt Liz? Treatment couldn't save her. I won't be able to manage.

Level of concern: 8/10

Potential thinking errors

(1) Mental filter/Tunnel vision: selective attention to one unfortunate health-related situation.

(2) Overgeneralization: making broad conclusions about all people facing cancer from one situation.

(3) Catastrophizing: assuming the worst-case scenario will happen in my situation (i.e. that I will get diagnosed with cancer, treatment will fail and I will die).

Actions taken or not taken (safety behaviors & avoidance)

(1) Excessive checking: I repeatedly gave myself thorough breast examinations throughout the day for several days.

(2) Reassurance seeking: I called my mom to talk for 45 minutes about my concern. I gathered detailed information about my aunt's diagnosis as well as asked her repeatedly if she thought I had cancer too.

Potential underlying core beliefs behind health concerns

(1) Overestimating likelihood/severity of health problems: inflating the odds that the breast pain is cancer when there are more likely explanations (i.e. overestimating probability). Also, assuming that I will not only be diagnosed with cancer but that treatment will be ineffective (i.e. overestimating severity).

(2) Vulnerability to sickness and inability to cope: I am assuming that if I did get diagnosed with cancer, I would be as good as dead. I assume my body is weak and unable to cope with a disease.

(3) Inadequacy of medical resources: I am automatically assuming that, even if I did have cancer, physicians and tests won't be able to detect it in time or treat it.

Date & situation or trigger & anxiety level (0–10)

August 27

I have been feeling more tired lately. After finding no major concerns in bloodwork and other tests, doctors recommended I get more exercise and eat healthier food and take a vitamin supplement

Anxiety: 9/10

Automatic thought about the situation & level of concern (0–10)

It is unacceptable that these doctors and tests can't find a clear explanation for my fatigue. Something is seriously wrong with me. I can feel it.

Level of concern: 9.5/10

Potential thinking errors

(1) Unrealistic expectations: I'm assuming that doctors/tests should be able to give me an explanation about any symptom I have with 100 percent certainty.

(2) Emotional reasoning: assuming that something is wrong with my health just because I am anxious about it.

Actions taken or not taken (safety behaviors & avoidance)

Reassurance seeking: I went to three different doctors to try to get the answers I was looking for. I read incessantly about causes of fatigue online.

Potential underlying core beliefs behind health concerns.

(1) Rigid health beliefs: I am assuming that to be healthy, I can't have any symptoms. Thus, having the symptom of fatigue is automatically a serious problem.

(2) Inadequacy of medical resources: I am assuming that medical resources are insufficient simply because they cannot tell me the cause of my symptom.

References

1 Shi C, Du X, Chen W, Ren Z. Predictive roles of cognitive biases in health anxiety: A machine learning approach. *Stress and Health*. Published online August 10, 2024. <https://doi.org/10.1002/smi.3463>

2 Du X, Witthöft M, Zhang T, Shi C, Ren Z. Interpretation bias in health anxiety: A systematic review and meta-analysis. *Psychological Medicine*. Published online November 9, 2022:1–12. <https://doi.org/10.1017/s0033291722003427>

3 Gessner J, Schulz JO, Melzig CA, Benke C. Role of interoceptive fear and maladaptive attention and behaviors in the escalation of psychopathology – a network analysis. *Cognitive Behaviour Therapy*. Published online April 9, 2024:1–20. <https://doi.org/10.1080/16506073.2024.2336036>

4 Olatunji BO, Deacon BJ, Abramowitz JS, Valentiner DP. Body Vigilance in nonclinical and anxiety disorder samples: Structure, correlates, and prediction of health concerns. *Behavior Therapy*. 2007;38(4):392–401. <https://doi.org/10.1016/j.beth.2006.09.002>

5 Salkovskis P, Warwick H. Meaning, misinterpretations, and medicine: A cognitive-behavioral approach to understanding health anxiety and hypochondriasis. In: V Starcevic and DR Lipsitt, eds. *Hypochondriasis: Modern Perspectives on an Ancient Malady.* Oxford University Press; 2001;202–222. <https://psycnet.apa.org/record/2001-00239-009>

6 Marcus DK, Gurley JR, Marchi MM, Bauer C. Cognitive and perceptual variables in hypochondriasis and health anxiety: A systematic review. *Clinical Psychology Review.* 2007;27(2):127–139. <https://doi.org/10.1016/j.cpr.2006.09.003>

7 Abramowitz J, Braddock A. *Psychological Treatment of Health Anxiety and Hypochondriasis: A Biopsychosocial Approach.* Accessed August 27, 2024. <https://pubengine2.s3.eu-central-1.amazonaws.com/previewith99.110005/9781616763473_preview.pdf>

8 Fergus T, Asmundson G. Cognitive and behavioral mechanisms of health anxiety. In: Hedman-Lagerlof E, ed. *The Clinician's Guide to Treating Health Anxiety: Diagnosis, Mechanisms, and Effective Treatment.* Elsevier Academic Press; 2019:43–64. <https://psycnet.apa.org/record/2019-25905-004>

3

Reduce estimation errors

People with health anxiety tend to assume that disease is more *common* and more *severe* than it actually is, statistically speaking. This is often referred to as the 'overestimation of threat,' 'threat bias' or 'threat misappraisal.' In this chapter, we are going to critically examine the assumption that serious disease is *common* to help you start to think of the odds more accurately. In the next chapter, we will tackle the assumption about disease *severity* or that getting diagnosed with a disease would automatically result in the worst-case scenario.

My client Kylie had an ongoing fear of having multiple sclerosis. Anytime she noticed tingling in her foot or leg, felt weak or was clumsy in some way, she would spiral and imagine herself living with and dying from MS. I got the sense from our conversations that she was inflating the likelihood of this happening to her so I asked for her thoughts on her chances. Off the top of her head, she guesstimated that she had about a 15 percent chance of getting MS. In reality, she had a 3 in 1,000 or less than half of 1 percent chance of developing MS.[1]

Further, Kylie didn't know her biological father, and she believed this unknown factor increased her odds of having MS. After all, she rationalized that this man *could* have MS and, if he did, she would be highly likely to get it. Again, we examined her estimates more closely and she guessed that if her biological father had MS, she would have a 35–40 percent chance of getting MS. In reality, *even in the unlikely event* that he had this disease, her risk of developing MS would increase from <0.5 percent to 3–4 percent.[1] Indeed, there is an increased risk but nowhere near what Kylie was assuming.

I have had these types of conversations with clients time and time again. Whatever the feared disease is: Lyme disease, early-onset dementia, HIV, bacterial meningitis, Parkinson's, cancer. I have seen clients overestimate their odds of having a wide variety of diseases. They weren't intentionally overestimating the odds, of course. They were often just making hasty ballpark estimates without thinking too much about it and did not challenge their assumptions by looking at the actual data.

Inflating the odds when you have a medical condition

If you have a diagnosed medical condition, this chapter might seem irrelevant to you. After all, you did in fact get diagnosed with something and, therefore, are among those who 'beat the odds' so to speak. While this is true, there are other ways people with health anxiety make estimation errors. We can overestimate the likelihood that a symptom is an urgent or serious concern as well as underestimate the likelihood of a symptom being due to something minor or benign.

If you suffer from health anxiety while living with a medical condition, symptoms can be particularly distressing. It can be easy to develop a habit of assuming that all bodily sensations and symptoms indicate your medical condition is worsening (or returning). However, your body is still a normal human body that produces symptoms for a variety of reasons. Thus, the techniques in this chapter may help you to learn how to not overestimate the likelihood that bodily sensations and symptoms automatically signal a crisis or urgent concern related to your medical condition.

Dysfunctional beliefs and biased information processing

When you believe getting diagnosed with a serious or terminal illness is a common experience, you pay selective attention to any 'evidence' in your environment that proves this to be true.[2] Your ears might perk up anytime you hear names of certain diseases. You might immediately stop scrolling on social media if a video or post pops up about someone getting diagnosed with cancer. Or you might easily recall the memory about an acquaintance from high school who suddenly died from a brain aneurysm at 28.

These are examples of information processing biases and, over time, they strengthen your belief that serious disease is everywhere. Eventually, you become convinced that you are just waiting to join the rest of society and be taken down by a serious or terminal illness. How could you not think this way? When you drown yourself in the concept of illness and disease and pay little attention to all the cues of health and wellness that surround you every day, sickness is most certainly going to seem more prevalent.

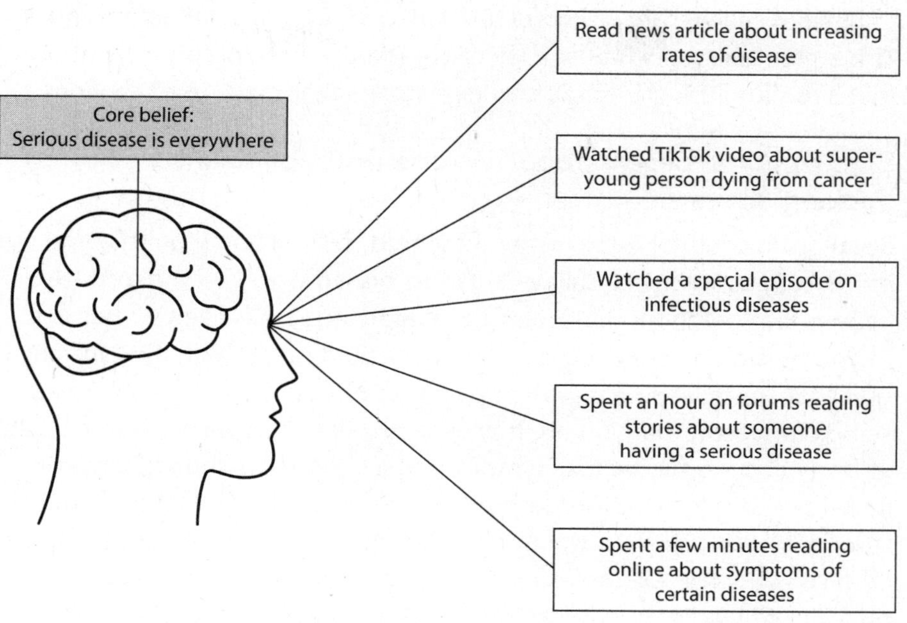
Core belief:
Serious disease is everywhere
Read news article about increasing rates of disease
Watched TikTok video about super-young person dying from cancer
Watched a special episode on infectious diseases
Spent an hour on forums reading stories about someone having a serious disease
Spent a few minutes reading online about symptoms of certain diseases

Serious disease is everywhere

One of my biggest fears has always been getting diagnosed with cancer. I mean, I had dabbled in the fear of other types of diseases, sure. But *cancer*. Even seeing or hearing the word alone could send me right over the edge. And, of course, it seemed like cancer stories followed me everywhere. My close friend. My great grandmother. My husband's coworker's nephew. The one guy at the hair salon. That tragic post on Facebook. All those characters with cancer on *The Other Sister*, *50/50*, *A Walk to Remember*, *The Fault in Our Stars* and all the other cancer movies I had watched. After years of drowning myself in stories of illness and death, I eventually accepted that cancer, and terminal illnesses in general, were lurking, just waiting to pounce on me. Of course, I now know that serious disease only seemed more prevalent because I paid selective attention to illness- and death-related content.

While I was busy seeking out stories about sickness, I was simultaneously paying very little attention to all of the cues of health and wellness in my environment that surrounded me every day. And this is, unfortunately, easy to do. Healthy stories just aren't talked about or noticed as much because they are not as interesting. Think about it this way: would you ever hear someone say, '*Hey, you know my friend*

Chris from college? He is 40 and has three kids and has not gotten cancer.' This statement sounds absurd because there is nothing unusual about that situation. It is the tragic and rare stories that make the headlines.

Dysfunctional beliefs about disease probability and thinking errors

Recall from Chapter 2 that when you hold dysfunctional beliefs, you are more likely to interpret daily events in a biased way. If you genuinely believe that getting a debilitating or deadly disease is likely to happen to you, it is completely logical that you would be on high alert for any sign that some terrible disease is going to gobble you up soon. Thus, it stands to reason that you are going to suspect every lump, bump, scab or body ache to be the first symptom of a serious diagnosis. Similarly, it makes sense for you to interpret external events (e.g. a scary health story, a phone call from the nurse) as a sign of your impending demise. I'll give you a few examples of how the overestimation of serious disease can lead you to interpret events in a biased way.

Jumping to conclusions: Making assumptions about the likelihood of having or getting a disease with little or no evidence.

During my youth and early adulthood, I was terrified of contracting HIV. In my life I have probably had over 15 HIV tests, even though I wasn't engaging in risky behaviors. One time I was in the waiting room at the doctor's office, awaiting blood work results from a routine physical, which included, per my request, an HIV test. The nurse called my name and I followed her back to a little office. As I entered the room, she glanced up from her clipboard and did not smile. At that moment, I *knew*. She was about to tell me I had tested positive for HIV. Clearly, she was not smiling at me because she was judging me for whatever I might have done to contract it. Overwhelmed, I burst into tears. Her facial expression immediately transformed into one of curiosity and compassion. '*Honey, are you okay?*' I explained what was wrong as I wiped my tears.

She quickly assured me that all of my bloodwork results looked great and I did not have HIV. The only issue she meant to raise was that my cholesterol was slightly high and she wanted to discuss some diet and exercise recommendations to improve it. If I had waited just a couple more minutes instead of jumping to conclusions and attempting to read the nurse's mind, I could have spared us both the drama. Instead, because I was overestimating the likelihood of me having HIV, I took a tiny (and irrelevant) piece of information and made a drastic and inaccurate conclusion.

Mental filter or Tunnel vision: focusing only on the facts that support your belief that serious disease is common, while ignoring or dismissing the other facts that do not support this belief.

My client, Jim, got the results back from his annual physical and it showed that, overall, all of his levels were in the 'normal' range and there were no major concerns. The only minor issue that the doctor discussed with him was that his LDL cholesterol was slightly elevated. His physician didn't believe medication was necessary at that point but recommended a few lifestyle changes (exercise, diet). Jim and his doctor made a plan for him to return at a later date to see if the lifestyle changes made a difference in his LDL levels.

Jim struggled with these results because he was convinced that his cholesterol would inevitably lead to heart disease, which would then lead to a heart attack or stroke. In the days and weeks that followed getting this information, he became progressively more fearful of having a sudden cardiac event. He started to revert to old habits of checking his pulse regularly throughout the day and refraining from doing any activity that would elevate his heart rate. Essentially, Jim was hyper focused on the one piece of 'threatening' information that supported his belief that he was likely to die young from a heart attack and was filtering out all of the other information that showed he was, overall, in good physical health.

Overgeneralization: making a broad, negative conclusion about the overall likelihood of getting a disease based on one or a few health-related events.

Many years ago, I learned that a friend's cousin in her thirties, with two young children, was diagnosed with Stage 4 colon cancer. I lost it. I thought, *See? This is exactly the kind of thing I am afraid will happen to me. And, clearly, it does happen. So what if I'm next?* My health anxiety surged that week, and I vigilantly searched for any gastrointestinal symptoms that could possibly point to colon cancer.

Now this specific fear of colon cancer eventually faded. But the tragic story about a young mother with late-stage cancer perpetually loomed over me. Every time a new potential health threat emerged, that sad story, and others like it, reminded me that I wasn't crazy to expect this type of diagnosis could happen to me. Essentially, I took a single, sad story and drew broad conclusions about the likelihood of me (and others) having advanced colon cancer or some other devastating illness.

Let's show those numbers who's boss

So, how do we stop ourselves from inflating the numbers and assuming that serious diseases are lurking behind every corner? After all, if it were that easy, you would have done it already and wouldn't be reading this book. Several cognitive techniques can help you to take a step back and use logic to view your chances of getting a serious disease more realistically. We will start with the most general approach, using Socratic questions to challenge problematic thoughts.

Socratic dialogue

Socratic dialogue involves using a series of questions to help you evaluate and reconsider your assumptions and conclusions. These questions can help you harness critical thinking skills instead of automatically accepting all thoughts as facts. You are essentially teaching your brain to see health-related situations in new, more balanced and adaptive ways.

In Chapter 2, you learned about the different types of thinking errors related to health anxiety. Now, you are going to learn how to challenge these problematic thoughts. When we assume all of our thoughts are valid, we move through our day accepting them as facts and, thus, react to them as though they are facts. You notice a funny taste in your mouth and you recall a Facebook post about a family member who was diagnosed with a brain tumor after experiencing strange tastes and smells. You conclude that you have brain cancer and begin to experience the sadness and anger that accompany this new, presumed reality. The problem with this is that, in these situations, you spend a lot of time and energy reacting to fiction, causing unnecessary and preventable suffering.

Instead, we want you to learn how to critically evaluate and challenge distressing thoughts about your health to reframe any that are distorted. This is where Socratic questioning comes into play. Learning to question your assumptions will not only help you in the current, specific situation you are dealing with but also solidify long-term changes in how your brain seeks out and processes information. But you have to practice this skill. This is called *retraining or rewiring your brain*. Over time, you will interpret situations more accurately and adaptively and will be less likely to engage in thinking errors. I always tell my clients that my goal is for them to build their skill set so they can eventually become their own CBT therapist.

Let's start by helping you become familiar with Socratic questioning. Essentially, you'll want to ask yourself a series of open-ended questions that allow you to examine the evidence for your thoughts and challenge assumptions. In other words, you want to look for inconsistencies, contradictions, exceptions and find plausible alternative ways of viewing the situation. It is important to be curious, have an open mind and be honest with yourself throughout this process.

Engaging in Socratic dialogue may include a variety of questions. Below are examples that can help you begin to think differently about the likelihood of you having a serious disease or the likelihood that your disease is worsening or returning. Note that this is not an exhaustive list. Socratic dialogue is nuanced and will depend on your specific circumstances and thoughts. The point is to learn to think critically and consider alternative viewpoints. Again, the more you practice this, the more skilled you will become at thinking of relevant and helpful questions to ask yourself when you are challenging distressing thoughts.

Table 1 Examples of Socratic questions for overestimating likelihood of disease

- Are my predictions closer to the worst-case scenario or the best-case scenario? What could be the most likely scenario? Have my predictions been wrong in the past?
- Am I catastrophizing? Are there any potential benign, minor or otherwise non-catastrophic explanations for this symptom? For instance, could this symptom be due to anxiety or random 'body noise'?
- What is the evidence for me having X disease? Or what is the evidence that this symptom indicates my disease is progressing/worsening?
- Am I jumping to conclusions based on a small amount of evidence?
- How valid is this evidence? Are there biases/inaccurate assumptions?
- What is the evidence against me having X disease? Or what is the evidence against the idea that this symptom means my disease is progressing?
- Am I considering all of the evidence or just the evidence that supports my assumption or fear?
- What would I say to a friend if they had this symptom? Do I tend to see the likelihood of others having a serious disease more realistically than my own?
- Am I making connections that are not logical or that are based on magical thinking? How so?
- Am I assuming I am likely to have X disease because of how I am feeling? How so?
- What is the impact of me assuming every symptom is urgent or is due to a serious illness? What could be the impact of me assuming symptoms are due to something minor or benign?
- Am I hyper focusing on the rare, tragic stories about diseases and ignoring the more common stories about health? How so?
- Am I drawing general conclusions about the likelihood of me having a disease based on one or a couple of health-related situations? How so?

Practice makes perfect

Now, we will have you practice using these and other questions to reconsider your assumptions. Recall the thought record you completed in Chapter 2. This is an extension of that record, which also includes a section to challenge your thoughts with Socratic questions. Just like with the thought record in Chapter 2, you will identify the situation, thoughts, feelings and potential thinking errors. However, this time you will also begin to challenge these thoughts.

Review the list of common thinking errors:

1 Black-and-white thinking
2 Jumping to conclusions, including fortune telling and mind reading
3 Catastrophizing
4 Unrealistic expectations
5 Mental filter/tunnel vision
6 Emotional reasoning
7 Overgeneralization
8 Magical thinking

Next, see the extended thought record. This week, try to practice identifying situations, thoughts, feelings as well as challenging any thinking errors using the relevant Socratic questions listed above. Bonus points if you can come up with additional relevant questions or points to critically analyze and challenge your thoughts!

Thought record

Date & situation or trigger & level of anxiety (1–10)

September 10
Forgot the name of that kid's mom in my daughter's class.
Anxiety: 8/10

Automatic thought about the situation & level of concern (1–10)

How could I forget something like this? I just had a 20-minute conversation with her yesterday. This is what happens with Alzheimer's. You start forgetting small things at first, and then you get lost on your way home from work.

Level of concern: 9/10

Potential thinking errors

Jumping to conclusions: Assuming a symptom is due to a serious disease with little evidence.

Response to thoughts or challenging with Socratic dialogue

I am jumping to conclusions about having Alzheimer's based on one minor instance. There is no other evidence to suggest I have this disease. People forget for a variety of benign or minor reasons, such as stress, anxiety, depression, lack of sleep, medications and dehydration, most of which could explain me forgetting.

Date & situation or trigger & level of anxiety (1–10)

September 15

A colleague at work was just diagnosed with breast cancer.

Anxiety: 7/10

Automatic thought about the situation & level of concern (1–10)

Of course. This happens to so many people. It's only a matter of time. I could be next.

Level of concern: 7.5/10

Potential thinking errors

Overgeneralization: making general conclusions about the overall likelihood of serious disease based on one situation.

Response to thoughts or challenging with Socratic dialogue

It is very sad and unfortunate that my colleague got cancer but just because it happened to her doesn't mean it will happen to me. The vast majority of people in my life are not living with cancer. It makes me anxious to see her dealing with this and my anxiety is making me see the situation as a threat to my health when it is not.

Absolute risk versus relative risk

In the digital age we live in, we are continually bombarded with health-related information. It is, therefore, crucial that we understand the difference between absolute and relative statistics. You can probably recall times when you have seen a headline that says something like, '*If you eat this, you are 10x more likely to develop cancer.*' In these cases, they are reporting 'relative risk.' Unfortunately, reporting *only* the relative risk can be misleading. I'll explain.

The 'absolute risk' of a disease is your risk of developing a disease over a period of time. We all have an absolute risk of developing a certain disease. This can be expressed as: '*you have a 1 in 10 risk of developing X disease*' or, put another way, '*you have a 10 percent chance of developing X disease.*' Relative risk, on the other hand, is used to compare the risk in two different groups of people. For example, you could be comparing people who work out versus people who don't work out or smokers versus non-smokers. This would be expressed as: *'people who smoke are X times more likely to develop X disease than those who don't smoke.'*

When you only know the relative risk, the numbers are essentially meaningless. Think about it this way: if I told you I have twice as much money in my bank account as my brother, that information really tells you nothing about the amount of money I have until you know what my brother has—if he has 20 dollars in the bank, then I have 40 dollars in the bank. If he has 200,000 in the bank, well, then I have 400,000 in the bank. You get the picture.

Given that the media often emphasizes relative risk, it is important to gather all the facts about it. For example, a widely reported study was published indicating that multiple childhood CT scans could triple the risk of brain cancer or leukemia. However, the absolute risk was much smaller: one additional case of a brain tumor and one additional case of leukemia per 10,000 children.[3] Of course, this is still concerning and these scans would only make sense if the benefits of undergoing a scan outweigh the risks. However, knowing only the relative risk sounds much more alarming.

The simple takeaway message is to use discernment when you consume health-related content. Check to see if they also report the absolute risk, as they should. If they do, take a look at the numbers and use them to help put this new information into perspective. *You need all the facts.* If you only read the frightening headline and simply move on with your day, you may be inadvertently adding to your health anxiety and further reinforcing problematic beliefs about health.

Examine the evidence for thoughts

Examining the evidence is a detailed exercise to help you examine the validity of a given thought. It is a great technique to help you challenge any type of anxious thought, including anxious thoughts about your health. This technique is a more in-depth version of one of the commonly used Socratic questions. It gives you the opportunity to pull back and take a 'helicopter view' of the situation so that you can see all of the evidence *for* and *against* your thought in one place. Now, let me tell you a little story about my lung cancer 'scare.'

When I was 21 and a senior in college, I had my first cigarette. I blame my roommate. One of our favorite activities to do on study breaks or after drinking was to sit out on our balcony and have stimulating, often philosophical conversations. During these little chats, she smoked and I didn't. Until one night, I did. It tasted like I imagined it would if I had licked the bottom of a soupy garbage can. But the slight buzz I got from it felt great. And, as dumb as it sounds now, holding that cigarette while talking about psychology and politics made me feel like an intellectual.

Well, as you might suspect, this once-a-week engagement snowballed. Cigarettes went with me everywhere. I would throw out my fresh pack, quit for a few months, buy a new pack and start back up, only to quit yet again. After two years of this nonsense, I decided enough was enough and I never looked back.

Little did I know, these smoking escapades would haunt me for many years to come. Images of me bent over in a hospital bed, coughing up blood and gasping for breath, have flooded my mind on many occasions. For years, I provided counseling to patients on hospice, a couple of whom actually died of lung cancer right in front of me. I was profoundly affected by some of these situations. *This is going to be me.*

About six years ago, I was walking up the staircase in my house and I had to catch my breath when I got to the top. Huh, that is weird. Why would I be out of breath from—*uh oh.* It hit me. This was it. My time had come. Of course, I immediately pulled my phone out and began the (very sensible) Google search: shortness of breath AND lung cancer. I was instantly flooded with information from the American Cancer Society to every medical website that ever existed, all talking about shortness of breath being one of the key symptoms of lung cancer.

Well, shame on me for engaging in this safety behavior. As I mentioned, this was only six years ago. I knew better than this, dammit! Even today, I slip up at times and revert to old habits. Still, thanks to the skills I had in my toolbox, when I noticed myself heading down that same ol' rabbit hole with lung cancer, I was able to stop and climb back out. First, I considered whether these thoughts about my having lung cancer could be distorted in some way. Big reveal: they were definitely distorted. I was both *jumping to conclusions* and *catastrophizing*. Next, I began to examine the evidence for this thought.

Example of the 'Examine the Evidence' exercise

This strategy is used to evaluate specific thoughts or beliefs to better understand the accuracy of specific thoughts and beliefs. Remember, the whole goal of CBT is not *positive thinking* but realistic and logical thinking. And, because our anxious minds can lead us to overestimate the probability and severity of a threat, it is critically important to put these thoughts to the test. Think of yourself as a scientist who is collecting data. Review a brief explanation of how to do this exercise below.

- Open up a Google Doc or take a piece of paper and create a table with two columns:
  - evidence *for* the thought
  - evidence *against* the thought
- Identify the anxious thought and write it down. Be as specific as possible.
- Assess the extent to which you believe this thought (on a scale of 0–100).
- Collect the evidence *for* your anxious thought (e.g. in my case, that shortness of breath is the first sign of lung cancer).
- Collect the evidence *against* the thought (e.g. the evidence that shows my shortness of breath is not lung cancer).
- Return to the evidence *for* the thought section and reframe or challenge any 'evidence' that seems biased or inaccurate. Note, this is an important step because your anxiety may be leading you to believe something is 'evidence' when it isn't and you need to give yourself the opportunity to challenge it. It can be helpful to write or type the reframes in a different color (I prefer red). This helps you to recognize the distinction between the evidence *for* the anxious thought and your reframes or arguments *against* any biases in your evidence for the anxious thought. I find making this distinction particularly useful when we go back to review all of the data together.
- Review all of the evidence together and reassess the extent to which you believe your distressing thought. This allows us to see whether the exercise was helpful at all. It doesn't need to be drastic. Even a reduction by ten points might make you feel less anxious.
- Identify a few alternative explanations for the symptom.

Anxious thought: *This shortness of breath is the first sign of lung cancer.*

Degree of belief before the exercise (0–100): **70/100**

Degree of belief after the exercise (0–100): **45/100**

Table 2 Evidence around the anxious thought

Evidence FOR the thought	Evidence AGAINST the thought
• I smoked on and off for about two years. *Reframe: Yes, it is possible this leads to cancer. I am probably more likely to get cancer than someone who never smoked. However, I only smoked on and off for a two-year period and haven't smoked anything in over 15 years so that at least decreases the odds.* • Both of my dad's parents died of lung cancer at age 60. *Reframe: They both chain-smoked for 40+ years, to the point that the walls in their house turned puke yellow.* • I partied and was irresponsible when I was younger so this would be payback for my poor choices. *Reframe: This is superstitious nonsense. Karma does not determine who lives or dies. Biology and environment are influential factors, not misdeeds.* • I just have a feeling it is cancer—something feels 'off' in that area of my body. *Reframe: This is emotional reasoning and it is a thinking error. In the past I have often 'felt' like I have a serious disease simply because of my anxiety and, consequently, my tendency to overestimate the likelihood of a threat.* • Lots of people die of lung cancer every year. I have heard stories about people getting cancer even though they never smoked or didn't smoke for a really long time. *Reframe: It is possible that I have cancer because I smoked for two years. But if I am going to consider this, I must also consider all of the people who don't die from lung cancer who smoked at some point in their life. I am more likely to pay attention to the surprising stories about people who didn't smoke or smoked a short time and got cancer. I am less likely to notice the many other stories about people who didn't get lung cancer. Also, lifestyle is a huge contributing factor but biology (genetics specifically) can play a role with certain types of lung cancer and may have been a part of the stories I've heard. I don't know all the facts about these stories I have heard.*	• I have never had any concerns about my lungs in my life and have never been told of concerns about my lungs during any of my regular physicals (or during any other doctor appointment I have had). • I have no other symptoms of lung cancer, such as coughing excessively or coughing up blood, fluid-filled lungs, repeat infections, back pain, etc. Shortness of breath is the only symptom and there are many potential explanations. • I haven't smoked a cigarette in almost 15 years. During the only two-year period I smoked in my early twenties, it was on and off for brief periods of time. • The first time I felt shortness of breath was after I had walked up a flight of stairs. The fact that I am ridiculously out of shape is a more likely cause than cancer. Also, after I started to fear it was cancer, I experienced a lot of anxiety. Shortness of breath is a common anxiety symptom for me. I also kept hyper focusing on my breathing and, thus, was selectively attending to any 'cues' of shortness of breath. So, my anxiety and my selective attention were making my shortness of breath 'symptom' seem that much more pronounced. • There are lots of minor or benign explanations for shortness of breath that aren't related to serious diseases (e.g. being out of shape, asthma, low blood pressure, anxiety or other types of emotional distress). • Overall, I live a relatively healthy lifestyle. I tend to work out regularly (well, not lately but usually) and eat a nutritious, well-balanced diet. I also attend all recommended routine medical appointments and check-ups as well as take my vitamins. • Other than my paternal grandparents, there is almost no cancer in my family tree. Most of my relatives are living or have lived long lives. If they did die, it was an accident of some kind (i.e. my mom) or decades of drug abuse and alcoholism (i.e. my dad). Most of my grandparents/great grandparents lived into their nineties.

As a final step, I want you to ask yourself: Is there an alternative way of seeing the situation? There are usually a number of potential non-catastrophic explanations for your symptoms. However, in an anxious state, we often don't even consider these. A great new habit to develop is to consider as many potential non-catastrophic explanations as you can think of and even try to conjure up evidence for them. Think about how skilled you probably are at seeking out the threat. Use that talent in a new way!

In my case, the non-catastrophic explanations for symptoms include:

1 the impact of running up the stairs too quickly and being out of shape (perhaps the most obvious)
2 fatigue
3 not eating enough that day
4 anxiety
5 lack of sleep from having a newborn
6 anemia

Overall, the 'examine the evidence' exercise helped me to see the alleged threat a bit more realistically. Yes, it is possible that my shortness of breath was, indeed, the first symptom of lung cancer. It is also possible that tonight I slip, hit my head and drown in the bath or that tomorrow I get shot while shopping in the toy aisle at the store. Many threats are possible but how many of them are probable? And seeing all of the evidence for and against my having lung cancer allows me to better grasp this low probability.

My clients and I whip out Google Docs regularly in sessions to examine the evidence. This is helpful to explore the likelihood of fears that stem from all types of anxiety. And on almost every occasion, we find that the 'evidence against' column looks robust and meaty, while the 'evidence for' column looks rather empty and hollow. Why? Because anxiety leads us to inflate the numbers!

Now, does this exercise guarantee that nothing is wrong? Of course not. There are no guarantees in this uncertain world. But in most cases, exercises like these will help you see the low probability that your symptom is indicative of a serious or terminal illness. That said, if the concerning symptom or bodily sensations continue, worsen or new symptoms emerge, then it is best to take the necessary, *reasonable steps* to address it (e.g. consult with a doctor, get an exam, scan or physical of some kind). Otherwise, I hope you will use the data you derive from using this exercise to help you see your perceived problem a bit more realistically.

The 'Pie Chart' technique

One technique to help you more realistically estimate the probability of serious disease (or worsening disease) is the Pie Chart (or Bar Graph) technique.[4] Let's say you have a stomachache. You go to the doctor and, despite the doctor's belief that it is likely due to a virus, indigestion, or something else benign, you worry that it might be something much more serious, such as some type of cancer. You could use this technique to create a visual representation of the likelihood of a given symptom being a serious or terminal illness compared to the likelihood of the symptom being a result of something minor or benign.

First, we include three serious illness categories:

- illnesses that one could be cured from or experience a full recovery
- illnesses that are chronic but manageable
- terminal illnesses.

We then assign a small percentage to each of these three serious illness categories because we know those are much less likely than the benign or minor illness categories, statistically speaking.

For the remainder of the pie chart, come up with several potential non-catastrophic explanations for the symptom or bodily sensation. In this case, some potential minor explanations could include inflammation or an infection, diet-related, or menstruation-related.

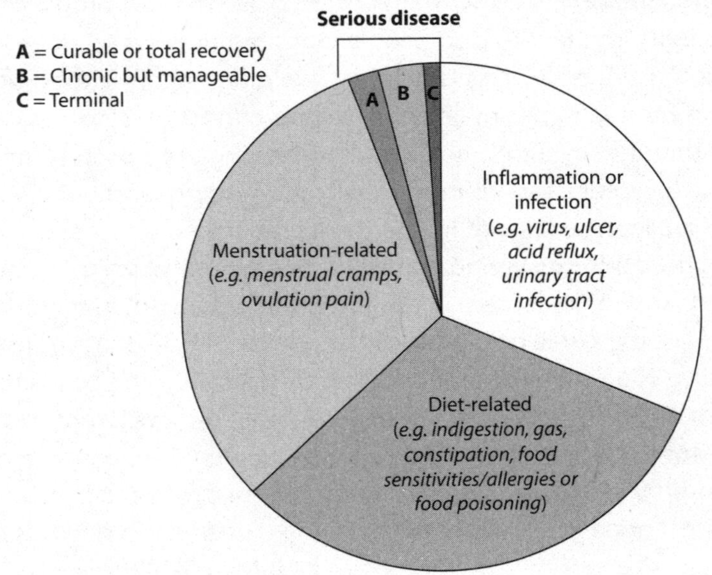

Now, looking at this figure, you can see that only one of the three serious illness categories involves a catastrophic outcome, which is the terminal illness subcategory. Even the other two serious illness categories (i.e. illnesses with full recovery or those that are chronic but manageable) are ultimately not catastrophic because you would be able to overcome or manage those illnesses.

The goal of this exercise is to help you recognize how easy it can be to overestimate how much of the graph represents the catastrophic outcome. Instead of it being just a small portion like it is in the pie chart above, in our mind, it often looks very different (see below). I know for me, when I had a symptom, I automatically assumed it was, more or less, just as likely to be due to a serious illness as it was a minor illness.

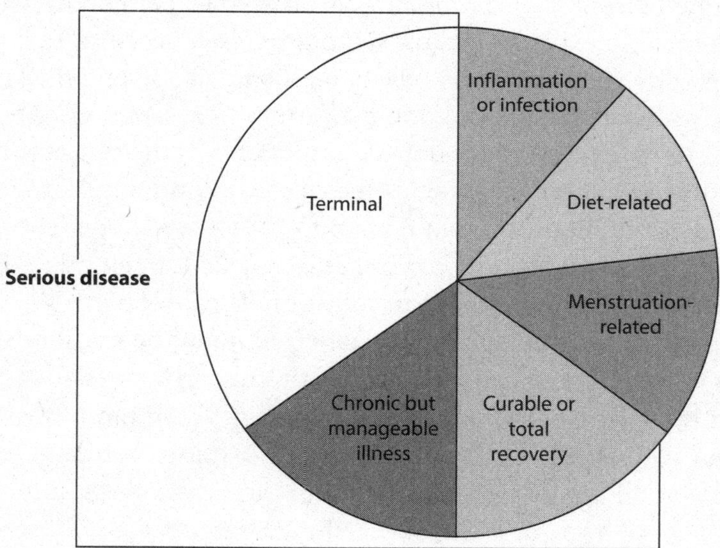

The Pie Chart technique can be helpful in a couple of ways. First, it can help you to build the habit of reflecting on and considering the wide range of non-catastrophic explanations for a symptom. It can also help you to realistically estimate the probability of you experiencing a catastrophic health outcome, which, again, is likely much lower than you assume it is.[4]

Completing your pie chart

The next time you feel anxious about a new symptom or bodily sensation, try this technique. When you complete your own pie chart, keep the following guidelines in mind. Start by listing out the serious illness categories in your pie chart. However, don't go into detail with these categories. Listing out all of the potential serious diseases could send you down a rabbit hole, which would be completely counterproductive. We are trying to move you *away from* ruminating on all of the catastrophic possibilities.

Next, consider all of the non-catastrophic explanations for your symptoms. This will take more time because these outcomes are much more likely and, thus, will consume a much bigger portion of your pie chart. Try to come up with a few key categories and then fill in those categories with as many different possibilities as you can.

Please note that, unless you have a medical background or knowledge in this area, you might need assistance coming up with possible medical explanations for symptoms. One option is to consult with someone you know who has medical knowledge and may be able to quickly offer some benign, non-catastrophic explanations. Another option is to search online for non-serious causes of the symptom just to get some ideas from reputable websites. If you do this, however, proceed with caution. You might want to have a loved one help you with this task or do this task for you, as it may be too tempting to go to the dark side and browse through catastrophic causes.

Also, if this task seems too intimidating to do in the midst of stressing about a new symptom, you can modify this to make it easier. Instead of using this exercise right after you notice a new symptom, you can test it out with an old situation that no longer makes you feel anxious. Perhaps you no longer feel anxious about the situation because the symptom went away or it was successfully treated by your doctor. This allows you to practice this new skill with a less anxiety-provoking situation, since you no longer fear the symptom. You can use this as a baby step to build confidence and, subsequently, take the next step of using it when you are anxious after noticing a brand new symptom.

Content cleanse

Recall that earlier we talked about when we hold a belief, we selectively attend to information that confirms this belief. When we believe serious disease is everywhere, we tend to search for data that confirms this. One strategy to improve this tendency is what I like to call a 'content cleanse.' We want you to be intentional about *limiting* the content you consume and what you surround yourself with every day.

It is important to note that there are situations that we cannot avoid, such as when a loved one gets sick or dies or when we work in certain environments, like a medical setting. Yes, people get sick and informative/reputable news articles about health/disease are necessary to read at times. However, in some areas of our lives we can exercise control by limiting the content we consume. For example, perhaps you didn't need to watch three Instagram reels in one week about someone with a terminal illness.

We will start by being proactive about the areas in your life that you can control. Think of this strategy as a way to protect that beautiful, imaginative mind of yours. As a first step, take inventory of the different ways you consume this type of content on a regular basis. I will give you a few examples from my client, Anthony.

- Reading stories about serious disease on Quora.
- Reading articles about people diagnosed with a serious or terminal illness.
- Watching videos on TikTok and Instagram about people's tragic personal stories with terminal disease.
- Reading comment sections in videos on social media, many people sharing the stories about people he knows getting a serious illness.
- Watching news clips or YouTube videos about people with serious diagnoses.
- Seeking out conversations with people at church or at work about people they know who have gotten a serious or terminal illness.

Once you have your list, think about how you might reduce or eliminate some of these behaviors. See detailed examples in the table below. After you identify your plan, select an accountability partner. Who already knows about this struggle of yours? Who is likely to encourage you to follow through with this task? After you come up with your plan, you are going to ask them for their help in holding you accountable. I recommend having them check in with you about it each week or every few days. Once you have selected someone, follow each of the steps in the worksheet below. Make sure to take the time to reflect on your experience in trying this technique.

Think of this as a small step you can take to develop more balanced and helpful beliefs about the likelihood of serious disease. Notably, clients have asked me if this exercise encourages avoidance of triggers and if, instead, it would be better to learn to deal with the triggers we face on a daily basis. I tell them, we are inevitably going to face situations at times that strengthen a given belief and trigger our health anxiety. If or when we face these situations, we must learn to deal with them productively, such as by incorporating them into our core belief system in an adaptive way.

This particular exercise addresses the issue of intentionally seeking out information for maladaptive beliefs. We aren't talking about everyday triggers but the issue of drowning yourself in specific content that supports your view, which creates a very biased and skewed depiction of reality. This exercise is to help develop a more balanced view of disease probability by not spending all your time on one side of the argument. Let's get started with an example.

Table 3 My content consumption limitation plan

Accountability partner: My wife				
Consumption behavior	Current frequency of this behavior	How this consumption behavior impacts me	Limitation plan	Ways that I will limit behavior or helpful steps I can take
Watching videos on Instagram and TikTok about people who have been diagnosed with a serious illness.	Lately, videos pop up on my feed (almost daily) and I usually watch the entire video (or most of the video) when they do pop up.	I've started to become convinced that serious disease at a young age is inevitable, which has increased my health anxiety. This has made every symptom and sensation seem very scary.	I will try to scroll past these videos whenever they pop up. I will also put other safeguards in place to prevent being inundated with videos like these.	*Safeguards:* I will click 'not interested' in the lower right-hand corner of the video and then click 'topic doesn't interest me' as the reason. I will click to block or mute the person (or hide the video) so that this and other similar videos don't show up in my feed.

Accountability partner: My wife				
Consumption behavior	Current frequency of this behavior	How this consumption behavior impacts me	Limitation plan	Ways that I will limit behavior or helpful steps I can take
Reading comment sections on social media videos.	I always read the comment sections of these kinds of videos. I like to see what people have to say about people they know who were diagnosed with the relevant disease.	It is completely overwhelming. It is one comment after another about people they know who have been diagnosed with various diseases. It scares me.	I will no longer read the comment section on health-related videos.	If I see these videos, I will scroll past. And I will not allow myself to click 'View comments.'

Table 4 Record of experiences in limiting content consumption

Consumption behavior plan	Log of experiences in limiting the behavior
Limiting watching videos on TikTok/Instagram	It was easy to do at first and fewer videos popped up after the first week because I had stopped watching them. But then over time I felt a desire to go back and watch these videos again. I started to worry that I was going to miss important information if I didn't follow people's accounts, especially those accounts that emphasize the 'first symptoms' they noticed before getting diagnosed. I went back and started watching again but then my wife helped me. She held me accountable, and I was able to refrain again. It has gotten better over time, and I am getting used to not watching these videos.
Refraining from reading comment sections	This was easier to follow through with. I did fail a couple of times. But soon after I started reading the comments, I was able to stop. I noticed right away the impact it was having on me. After failing a couple of times, I was able to completely refrain. It became easy just to keep scrolling and not click 'View comments.'

Reshaping your beliefs about disease probability

Up until this point, we have practiced challenging the estimation errors one makes when anxious about the cause of a symptom in day-to-day situations, such as through Socratic questioning, the 'examine the evidence activity' and the pie chart technique. Now, we will target the underlying core belief behind these estimation errors or thinking errors: the belief that getting a serious or terminal disease is probable. Recall that the thinking errors we have in our daily life result from having dysfunctional core beliefs about health and illness. In other words, we assume that a given symptom is likely due to a serious illness *because* we have the core belief that serious disease is more likely than it is.

It is, therefore, essential that we not only challenge our thinking errors but reshape the core beliefs behind these thinking errors. As discussed in Chapter 2, core beliefs play a large role in how we process information due to cognitive biases involved in how we collect and recall information. For example, we selectively attend to the data that supports our belief that serious or terminal disease is likely to happen to us and ignore data that does not support it. If we challenge the daily thinking errors but don't modify the belief itself, then we are merely putting a band aid on the proverbial wound. We will likely continue to make estimation errors and overestimate the likelihood that a symptom is due to a serious or terminal illness (or that a symptom suggests a medical condition is worsening).

You can challenge dysfunctional core beliefs by gathering evidence for and against the belief. This exercise can help you to interrupt your way of processing information and begin to process information in a new way. For example, in this case, it can help one to stop paying selective attention to information about the high likelihood of a serious or terminal illness and, instead, to begin to actively seek out information to support a more adaptive belief, that serious and terminal illnesses are not common, at least until late in life.

The core belief exercise

My client, Jarod, was experiencing a lot of health anxiety while attending medical school. He was in his mid-twenties and had no diagnosed medical conditions. He worried about having a sudden medical crisis, such as a heart attack, stroke or brain aneurysm. He was convinced that medical crises happened to young people often and lived in fear of it happening to him. We decided to explore this belief to take a deeper look at some of the reasons for his beliefs so we could challenge any that were based on faulty logic or inaccurate assumptions.

Below is the core belief exercise that Jarod and I completed together. First, read through the key steps on how to complete this exercise. There are also a few additional tips to keep in mind. Afterward, we will have you try this exercise with a core belief you have that is related to the likelihood of you getting a serious or terminal illness or having a sudden medical emergency. Below is a breakdown of the steps taken in this exercise to modify core beliefs.

Step 1: We write the maladaptive core belief at the top of the worksheet. In this case, *I am likely to get a serious illness or experience a sudden medical crisis because it is fairly common.*

Step 2: We then come up with a new, more adaptive belief. In this case, *I am unlikely to get a serious illness or have a sudden medical crisis at my age because it is rare.* The goal is for you to learn to believe this progressively more over time.

Step 3: We assess the degree to which you believe both beliefs (0–100, with 100 being the strongest). Remember, core beliefs are not permanent or static. They fluctuate depending on a variety of factors and can also change over time. This helps to highlight that important point.

Step 4: We make two columns, one to gather evidence for the old core belief and one to gather evidence for the new core belief.

Step 5: We begin collecting evidence for the old, maladaptive core belief.

Step 6: After we are finished, we go through the list of evidence and look for any potential thinking errors or inaccuracies. We write out the reframes next to each piece of evidence. Similar to the 'examine the evidence' exercise, it can be helpful to write or type the reframes in a different color (I prefer red). This helps you to recognize the distinction between the evidence *for* the dysfunctional core belief and your reframes or arguments *against* any biases in your pieces of evidence for that belief. I find making this distinction particularly useful when we go back to review all of the data together.

Step 7: We then move to the right side to list out all the evidence that contradicts the old core belief and appears to support the new core belief.

Step 8: We look through all of the evidence on both sides and then assess the extent to which you believe the old core belief as well as the extent to which you believe the new one. Please note that if you believe the new core belief even a tad more (and the old core belief a little less), I would conclude the intervention was helpful. Even a ten-point difference can improve your daily experiences to some extent.

Step 9: After you complete the exercise, continue collecting evidence on an ongoing basis.

Old core belief

I AM LIKELY TO GET A SERIOUS ILLNESS OR EXPERIENCE A SUDDEN MEDICAL CRISIS BECAUSE IT IS FAIRLY COMMON.

How much do you believe this core belief (*before the intervention*)? (0–100) **70**

EVIDENCE THAT SEEMS TO SUPPORT THE OLD CORE BELIEF (WITH REFRAME)

- In medical school, I am constantly flooded with examples of young people who get diagnosed with a serious or terminal illness or who have a sudden medical emergency, often with no history of health issues. *REFRAME: The examples discussed in medical school are chosen for a reason. Medical students learn from these situations. They are being trained to treat people with medical issues so, of course, the cases that are brought up involve people suffering from a serious disease or who are experiencing a medical crisis. Being in medical school can, inadvertently, give the false impression that serious medical crises are commonplace.*
- It seems that people get diagnosed with serious diseases all the time. I see videos on TikTok and Instagram about all these unsuspecting young people who get diagnosed with cancer or some other terminal illness. If it can happen to them, it can happen to me. *REFRAME: Social media is not a valid indicator of the distribution of a disease in the population. The algorithm feeds people what they like to watch. Although these awful situations do happen sometimes, these videos go viral because*

they are rare and intriguing or anxiety-provoking. The boring stories about people in decent health do not get nearly as much attention.

- Often, I have random concerns pop up with my body, such as pains, moles or skin blemishes or weird heart palpitations, which makes it seem more likely that there is something seriously wrong with me that has gone undiagnosed. *REFRAME: Aches and pains are often due to normal body noise. I have had doctors look at some symptoms and run relevant tests. I also go to my routine physicals and exams. So far, I have not been given any reason to think that the symptoms I have had are due to a serious or terminal illness. Also, I am often searching for symptoms to be worried about, which may lead me to hyper focus on the body noise and, thus, exacerbate the symptoms.*
- I was rebellious and irresponsible when I was younger, so I may get a disease as payback for my poor choices. *REFRAME: Unrelated events do not impact each other. I am not going to develop a disease because I didn't pay my parking tickets on time when I was young. That is superstitious, magical thinking.*
- I have heard there are rising cancer rates in the USA. *REFRAME: Although some evidence suggests an increase in cancer rates among certain types of cancers, the National Cancer Institute estimates that the age-adjusted rates for new cancer cases (of any site) remained stable from 2012–2021, while cancer-related deaths declined on average by 1.7 percent each year from 2013–2022.*[5]

How much do you believe this core belief (*after the intervention*)? (0–100) **45**

New core belief

I AM UNLIKELY TO GET A SERIOUS ILLNESS OR HAVE A SUDDEN MEDICAL CRISIS AT MY AGE BECAUSE IT IS RARE.

How much do you believe this core belief (*before the intervention*)? (0–100) **15**

EVIDENCE THAT CONTRADICTS THE OLD CORE BELIEF AND SUPPORTS THE NEW ONE

- I currently do not have any major underlying health conditions that might make me more susceptible to a sudden medical crisis or terminal illness. I haven't been sick with anything other than a cold, cough or some type of virus in years. Also, when I get my regular physicals, blood work and exams, most of it comes back as normal or at least with no major concerns.
- I am (relatively) young, and advanced age is the biggest risk factor for prevalent diseases in developed countries, such as cancer, cardiovascular diseases and neurodegenerative diseases.[6] Statistics show that diagnoses of serious diseases are extremely rare in my age group and are even unlikely in age groups that are older than mine.[7]
- I have a large social network of people in my past and present life, including family, extended relatives, friends, acquaintances, classmates, and colleagues. Many of these people I have known for decades. Among all of these people, it has been rare for me to know anyone with a life-threatening or terminal illness. This suggests that serious and terminal diseases are not as common as I am assuming.
- In 2021, the average life expectancy was 77.5 years in the United States,[7] which suggests the average person will not die from a terminal illness before this point. Although it does happen, the odds are in my favor.
- To my knowledge, I have pretty good genes in my family. I also take good care of my health. I exercise, eat well, get adequate sleep most nights, don't smoke and don't drink excessively. There is reason to believe that these factors could work in my favor in terms of reducing the likelihood of me developing or contracting a deadly illness or having a sudden medical crisis.
- Even if I were to have a disease, this does not mean it will be terminal. My chances of surviving the vast majority of illnesses are high, given my age, general decent health and the availability of medical treatments.

[*Note, this point will be discussed in great detail in the next chapter*].

How much do you believe this core belief (*after the intervention*)? (0–100) **75**

Once the exercise is over, you want to continue the habit of gathering evidence in this new way. With my clients, we usually add a section at the bottom of the table in each column that specifies 'this week's evidence.' Throughout their week, they seek evidence for their new belief. They also pay attention to anything they assume is evidence for their old belief, write that down and challenge it. This will help you continue the process of seeking and processing information in a new way.

Keep a few key points in mind when you are completing the core belief worksheet.

1 When you are identifying evidence for the old, maladaptive core belief, make sure you include everything. Even if you know the piece of evidence is silly, you still need to write it down. You want to give yourself the opportunity to challenge this and see how illogical it is. If you don't, you may continue to believe it to some extent, whether consciously or not.
2 Make sure you document the extent to which you believe both beliefs, before and after the intervention. This will help you to evaluate whether the intervention was helpful. Importantly, don't discount small changes in your belief after you do this. Even just a ten-point difference can help you feel better and means the intervention was useful to some degree.
3 You will not change your beliefs entirely during this one activity. Beliefs take time to change. Use this worksheet as a starting point. You will then work to build from there, slowly collecting evidence in your environment to support your new, healthy belief. In addition, you will want to continue to challenge any assumptions you make in your daily life that support your old belief.

In this chapter, you learned that people with health anxiety tend to overestimate the likelihood of serious disease and sudden medical crises or catastrophes. These beliefs develop from significant and meaningful experiences in our lives. They are then strengthened over time because of how we process information. Cognitive restructuring techniques can help you begin to critically examine your assumptions and reshape your thoughts and beliefs into those that are more adaptive.

Remember to practice using these techniques on a regular basis. Progress happens by making small changes in your thoughts and behaviors each day. You will likely not change your thinking if you merely read about these techniques or only try them once. It took you years to reinforce these beliefs and they are likely to be quite strong by now. It will take time and intentionality for you to change them. In the remaining chapters, you will continue practicing these skills to challenge different types of beliefs as well as to change unhelpful behaviors. If you commit to doing the work, you will notice a difference over time. Trust the process!

References

1 Hoff Communications. Who gets multiple sclerosis? MSAA. Published December 16, 2015.<https://mymsaa.org/ms-information/overviewwithwho-gets-ms/#:~:text=While%20MS%20is%20not%20contagious>

2 Shi C, Taylor S, Witthöft M, et al. Attentional bias toward health-threat in health anxiety: A systematic review and three-level meta-analysis. *Psychological Medicine*. 2022;52(4):604–613. <https://doi.org/10.1017/s0033291721005432>

3 Pearce MS, Salotti JA, Little MP, et al. Radiation exposure from CT scans in childhood and subsequent risk of leukaemia and brain tumours: A retrospective cohort study. The Lancet. 2012;380(9840):499–505. <https://doi.org/10.1016/s0140-6736(12)60815-0>

4 Taylor S, Asmundson GJG. *Treating Health Anxiety: A Cognitive-Behavioral Approach*. Guilford Press; 2004.

5 National Cancer Institute. Cancer of any site - cancer stat facts. SEER. Published 2018. <https://seer.cancer.gov/statfacts/html/all.html>

6 Niccoli T, Partridge L. Ageing as a risk factor for disease. *Current Biology*. 2012;22(17):R741–R752. <https://doi.org/10.1016/j.cub.2012.07.024>

7 Centers for Disease Control and Prevention. Life expectancy. Centers for Disease Control and Prevention. Published February 7, 2023. <https://www.cdc.gov/nchs/fastats/life-expectancy.htm>

4

Recognize ability to cope with disease

People with health anxiety not only overestimate the prevalence of serious disease but also overestimate how *severe* it will be if they do end up with a health condition. One reason they overestimate the severity of disease is because health-anxious people tend to assume they are weak and vulnerable. This assumption naturally increases the fear of disease because, if one believes they are particularly vulnerable, then it makes sense that they would assume that any disease could result in the worst-case scenario.

I struggled with the belief that I was weak and vulnerable for a long time. I'd bounce from one feared illness to another. I might fret for a few days that the scab on my hand was melanoma and, as that fear faded, a new fear would emerge that my sudden back pain was a sign of lung cancer. When I explored this tendency, I realized there was an underlying belief behind all of this illness-hopping. A big part of the reason I feared every potential disease was because I, mistakenly, saw myself as weak and fragile, as if I was just barely hanging on by a thread. My belief that I was weak led me to assume that any disease, big or small, would be life-threatening.

Another reason health-anxious people overestimate the severity of disease is because they tend to hold rigid beliefs about health and illness. They assume that health is dichotomous in that one is either healthy (and in the 'safe' zone) or they are sick (and in the 'danger' zone). Thus, if one has a diagnosed illness or fears that they do, they have entered the danger zone and, therefore, will inevitably face severe illness, likely resulting in the worst-case scenario.

I often fell prey to this type of rigid thinking. Once my physical results came back fine and with no concerns. I rejoiced the whole way home, bouncing along the highway and singing loudly, even welcoming a few extra cars into my lane. I felt fabulous. I mean, after all, I was in the 'healthy' category! But then later that same day, I noticed some redness in my eye and every ounce of joy drained from my body. In my mind, I had been demoted back down to the 'sickness' category or danger zone. With this new symptom came the assumption that I was no longer safe because if this symptom was, in fact, due to an underlying disease, it was likely to be severe and I would be doomed.

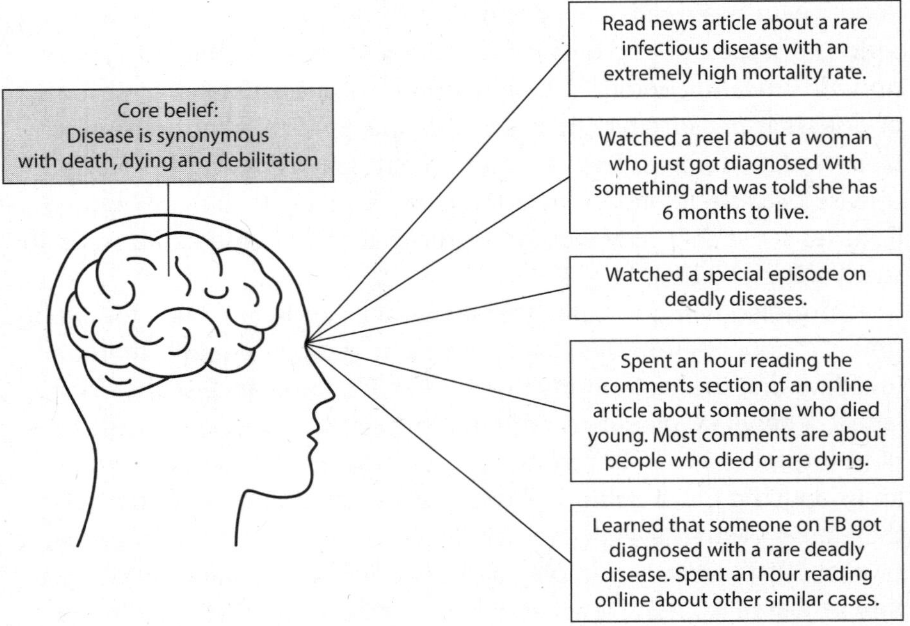

Core belief:
Disease is synonymous with death, dying and debilitation
Read news article about a rare infectious disease with an extremely high mortality rate.
Watched a reel about a woman who just got diagnosed with something and was told she has 6 months to live.
Watched a special episode on deadly diseases.
Spent an hour reading the comments section of an online article about someone who died young. Most comments are about people who died or are dying.
Learned that someone on FB got diagnosed with a rare deadly disease. Spent an hour reading online about other similar cases.

As discussed in Chapter 3, when we hold maladaptive beliefs, we search our environment for data that reinforces these beliefs. If you believe that disease is inevitably going to result in severe suffering, debilitation or death, you will pay selective attention to information in your environment that supports this belief. You might be quick to notice the stories about people who experience significant suffering and/or die, while paying less attention to the many stories of people who overcome an illness or who are managing it well. You also might vividly remember times when you struggled with an illness but have a harder time recalling times that you were ill but coped with it well.

Revising assumptions about disease severity

It is important to reconsider your assumptions about the severity of disease and be open to considering alternative views. Foremost, let me acknowledge that getting diagnosed with a disease can be extremely difficult, stressful and anxiety-provoking. And diseases can certainly be terminal. It is a basic fact of life that we will all face death at some point. Learning to live with this reality will be discussed thoroughly in a later chapter. However, despite all of this, it is essential to recognize that getting diagnosed with a medical condition is *not* synonymous with death and dying.

It is estimated that more than half of the US population lives with a chronic health condition, including arthritis, cancer, chronic obstructive pulmonary disease, coronary heart disease, asthma, diabetes, hepatitis, hypertension, stroke and weak or failing kidneys.[1] Although the rate of chronic disease is of grave concern, the increasing availability of effective treatments and improvements in disease prevention and detection make many chronic diseases preventable and/or treatable.[2,3,4] As a result of advances in modern medicine, the average life expectancy in the USA was 47 in 1900 and today it is almost 80.[5,6]

For a period of time while gaining my licensure hours, I worked in a hospital. At this point, my health anxiety was at a peak. You would think that working at a hospital, surrounded by patients with a wide variety of acute and chronic health conditions, would intensify my health anxiety. However, quite the opposite happened. My health anxiety improved because I started to see that one of my biggest fears, getting diagnosed with a medical condition, did not automatically translate to 'game over.' I found myself thinking, 'Wow, if they could survive that, with all their comorbidities, then maybe I would be okay if I had a health problem.'

Sure, I witnessed poor medical outcomes and that was difficult at times. However, I also worked with patients who had health conditions that were being effectively treated and, as a result, were stabilized or even improving. What's more, some of these patients came into the hospital with complicated medical histories and comorbidities and many of these situations were still managed well. That said, I know this is not the experience of everyone who works in a medical setting. Sometimes professionals in the medical setting experience a surge in health anxiety or find that it is triggered for the first time.

Perhaps a big reason why working in a hospital helped me was because it allowed me to witness the power of psychological and physical resilience as well as the adequacy of medical resources to help one cope with medical conditions. I began to see health as a spectrum, with many shades of gray, instead of black and white (i.e. healthy and 'safe' or sick and 'in danger'). I started to question my assumptions about being vulnerable and began to accept that, even if I were to get diagnosed with something, I would have options and would most likely be okay. Now, to be clear, at that point in my life I still had plenty of work to do to improve my health anxiety. But seeing evidence against this long-held maladaptive belief of mine was certainly a step in the right direction.

Dysfunctional beliefs about disease severity and thinking errors

As you know by now, holding the maladaptive belief about the severity of getting a disease can lead you to engage in thinking errors or to interpret everyday situations in a biased way. If you believe you are weak or vulnerable and, thus, assume that getting a diagnosis is the kiss of death, then it will inevitably influence how you interpret situations in your daily life. Below are a few examples of how beliefs that overestimate the severity of disease lead to biased interpretations.

Catastrophizing: Predicting only the most disastrous outcomes when it comes to your health. Any unexplained bodily sensation or symptom is a sign of disease and any disease would likely result in the worst-case scenario.

Catastrophizing is perhaps the most common, and most obvious, example of how assumptions about disease severity can lead to biased thinking. When I was a teenager, I saw a documentary that described people's experiences with psychosis. For the next week, I obsessively monitored my thoughts and searched for any 'signs' that I was experiencing psychosis, such as hallucinations or delusions. I vigilantly scanned my thoughts, terrified that if I was experiencing psychosis, it meant the end of my life—I would lose all ability to function normally and would no longer be 'me.' Of course, as per usual, I was overestimating how terrible it would be if I were to have a psychotic episode. Yes, these experiences can be awful but one can certainly still live a long and fulfilling life, even if they were to struggle with this.

All-or-nothing thinking: Viewing health in only two categories (i.e. perfect health or serious illness) instead of recognizing that health exists on a continuum. One assumes that having any disease automatically places them in the 'serious illness' category.

I had a client who had recently been diagnosed with type 2 diabetes. Understandably, this was extremely stressful, as she had to learn how to manage a health condition on top of already struggling with anxiety. When we explored what this diagnosis meant for her, we uncovered assumptions she had made about her life being 'over.' She expected that she would soon become debilitated by complications of diabetes and would not live long enough to see her adult children get married or have children. Although she was certainly facing a new challenge and she would need to make some potentially difficult lifestyle changes, including medication, diet and exercise, her life was not *over*. In today's world, people are able to live longer, healthier lives with diabetes. Instead of seeing herself as being overall healthy while facing a new health challenge, she saw herself as having made an irreversible switch from 'health status' to 'disease status.'

Mental filter or Tunnel vision: Focusing only on the facts that support your beliefs about the severity of disease, while ignoring or dismissing the other facts that do not support this belief.

One of my client's colleagues got diagnosed with breast cancer. This was a huge source of stress for my client, watching her colleague struggle through diagnosis and treatment. My client had always feared this would happen to her. When her colleague went into remission and was declared cancer-free, my client saw it as a miracle and talked about her colleague being one of the 'lucky few.' When we explored this further, my client revealed her assumption that when people get a serious diagnosis like cancer, it is almost inevitable that they will eventually succumb to it. Although it is unimaginably scary and difficult to face a serious disease like breast cancer, it is not rare to survive it. Data on women diagnosed with breast cancer between 2013 and 2019 suggests that the average five-year *relative* survival rate for all types of breast cancer is 91 percent (all stages combined). This means that women who have cancer are, on average, 91 percent as likely as women who don't have cancer to live for at least five years after diagnosis.[7] Obviously, the variance in outcomes depends on many factors, such as one's age and overall health, specific type of breast cancer, stage of cancer at diagnosis and response to treatment. However, it can point out the general truth that many women survive breast cancer.

Overgeneralization: Making a broad, negative conclusion about just how *bad* it will be to get diagnosed with something based on one or a few health-related events.

My grandma, completely unaware of how this would impact me, once told me a story about someone she knew who went to the dentist for a routine cleaning. This person was told by the dentist that she needed to see her doctor as soon as possible, due to some concerns he had about her teeth. She ended up having some type of late-stage cancer that had spread and was dead within weeks.

Of course, I had a million questions for my grandma about the details: '*Did she notice any other symptoms before going to the dentist? Had she noticed any issues with her teeth or gums or was this news to her? What type of cancer was it and where did it spread?*' My grandma didn't have any of these answers because the woman was merely an acquaintance. So, naturally, I decided to fill in the gaps with my own predictions. I concluded from this story that late-stage cancer could hit me at any time and then it would be 'lights out.'

This terrifying story colored my interpretations of my symptoms for months, even years after that conversation with my grandma. I'd discover a new symptom and think, *well, if I don't find out the answer for this symptom soon, I am going to end up just like the poor lady at the dentist*. I basically concluded that this case was likely to happen to any of us and, thus, we all needed to remain vigilant in order to save ourselves from a medical tragedy.

Socratic dialogue to challenge distortions about disease severity

In Chapter 3 you learned the rationale behind using Socratic dialogue to challenge problematic thoughts. This is a critical skill to develop so we will be exercising it in each chapter. In this chapter, you will learn how to use critical thinking to reframe how you see the severity (or 'badness') of getting a disease. If it helps, refresh your memory by reviewing the section in Chapter 3 on why and how using Socratic dialogue can have short- and long-term benefits in terms of how you see health and disease.

Remember, the goal of using these questions is to help you critically analyze your own thoughts and to look for inconsistencies, contradictions and exceptions to help you find new ways of viewing the situation. Try to explore your thoughts with a curious, open mind. Below is a list of several Socratic questions to help you assess whether getting a disease would be as horrifying as you might be assuming. Reflect on each of these questions and see what you come up with. Also, use these questions as inspiration to come up with your own.

Examples of Socratic questions related to *severity* of getting a disease:

- Am I hyper focusing on stories about people that were diagnosed with something and died? Am I considering all of the other stories about people who were diagnosed with a disease, serious or not, and were able to get treatment and recover or manage it well?
- Have I faced illnesses in the past? How was I able to overcome them?
- Do I know anyone in my personal life that has faced an illness and been able to cure it or treat it/manage it effectively?
- Am I drawing general conclusions about how bad it would be if I got a disease based on one or a few situations I have seen or heard of?
- Does my assumption represent black-and-white thinking (perfect health or serious illness)?
- Is there a more nuanced way of seeing this?
- What about all of the illnesses that are manageable or would fall in the middle of the spectrum (the middle of the two extremes)?
- How could I emotionally cope with this disease if I did have it? My social support system, personal resilience, faith, therapy, adaptive coping skills, support groups, self-help books, personal hobbies? Have any of these things helped me to cope with illness or other struggles in the past?
- How could I physically cope with this disease? What medical resources would allow me to manage, treat and/or overcome this disease or illness?
- What would it look like to cope and live well with this disease?
- Have I witnessed any examples of people in my life that have managed to cope with having a disease, physically and/or emotionally?
- If I did have X disease, am I overestimating the chances this will be incurable, debilitating and/or terminal?

Keep up the practice

Let's practice! Again, review the list of common thinking errors. For the next week, document your thoughts in a thought record. Any time you think you might be overestimating the severity or 'badness' of getting a disease, practice identifying thinking errors related to this. Next, challenge those thinking errors with the relevant Socratic questions above. I challenge you to practice coming up with your own questions as you see fit.

Review the list of common thinking errors:

1. Black-and-white thinking
2. Jumping to conclusions, including fortune telling and mind reading
3. Catastrophizing
4. Unrealistic expectations
5. Mental filter/Tunnel vision
6. Emotional reasoning
7. Overgeneralization
8. Magical thinking

Thought record

Date & situation or trigger & level of anxiety (1–10)

September 12

Missed a call from my doctor's office about the results of my physical

Anxiety: 9/10

Automatic thought about the situation & level of concern (1–10)

What if they are calling with bad news? I probably have diabetes, since it is in my family. I am going to die young from diabetes like my Aunt Sherry did and leave my kids motherless.

Level of concern: 9/10

Potential thinking errors

(1) Catastrophizing: predicting the most disastrous outcomes. I am assuming that having diabetes would automatically result in the worst-case scenario.

(2) Overgeneralization: making general conclusions about the severity of having diabetes based on my aunt's health outcomes.

Response to thoughts or challenging with Socratic dialogue

I am catastrophizing and assuming the absolute worst-case scenario if I were to get diagnosed with diabetes. Health is not a light switch: on or off. Even if I have diabetes, I would have treatments available to me to help me cope with it. I would also be able to make lifestyle changes. My aunt did not listen to what doctors recommended in her treatment plan. She continued to not take care of herself, which is why she did not survive. In addition to having medical resources, I would have a lot of support from my social network to help me cope with this diagnosis.

Date & situation or trigger & level of anxiety (1–10)

September 15

Spent a lot of time outside in the yard today.

Anxiety: 8/10

Automatic thought about the situation & level of concern (1–10)

What if I got bit by a tick? And then what if I get Lyme disease? Or worse, what if I don't find the tick bite so don't suspect I have Lyme disease or the doctors aren't vigilant and they might miss it and then I would end up with late-stage Lyme disease and have all of these health complications. My life would be ruined.

Level of concern: 7.5/10

Potential thinking errors

Catastrophizing: predicting the most disastrous outcomes. I am assuming that if I got bit by a tick, I would be likely to get Lyme disease from the tick. Also, I am predicting the worst-case scenario in that I either wouldn't notice or the doctors would miss the signs of me having Lyme disease, which would turn into a 'late-stage' situation with multiple health complications.

Response to thoughts or challenging with Socratic dialogue

I am assuming multiple worst-case scenarios at once. I am assuming that I would (a) get bit by a tick; (b) be among the 1–3 percent that would get Lyme disease from a tick bite; (c) miss the tick bite; and/or (d) doctors would miss signs of Lyme disease, which would then (e) turn into late-stage Lyme disease and my life would be difficult with multiple health complications. In reality, I most likely would not get bit by a tick that has Lyme disease and, even if I did, would likely see the bite and go and get antibiotics for it. Essentially, things would likely be fine.

Seeing health on a spectrum

Those of us with health anxiety can fall into the trap of thinking of health as dichotomous, in which we are either healthy and 'safe' or sick and 'in danger.' This leads us to assume that *any* health problem places us in the danger zone and is terminal or life-threatening. We therefore spend the majority of our time suffering in the danger zone, most likely unnecessarily. In reality, health, like many things in life, exists on a spectrum. In most cases, one is not either perfectly healthy or deathly ill. In between those two extremes are numerous other health situations or outcomes, the vast majority of which are treatable and manageable with disease management programs.

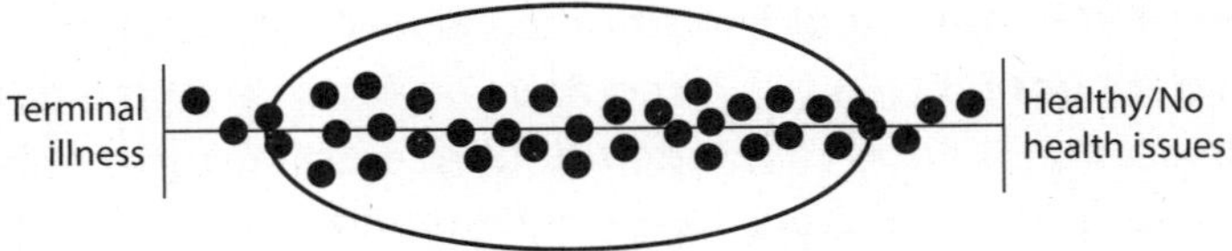

A client of mine, Erick, had an intense fear of dying from a heart attack. His dad died from a massive heart attack in his fifties. As Erick entered middle age, he became convinced that he would inevitably share the same fate as his father. His anxiety over this intensified as he climbed closer to the age of his father when he died.

Erick had been to his primary care doctor for routine physicals and had also undergone multiple heart tests, which came back 'normal' and did not reveal any signs of an issue. However, Erick did have high LDL cholesterol levels, which concerned him because it put him at higher risk for heart disease. Not surprisingly, Erick's fear of a heart attack led him to be hyper vigilant about symptoms related to breathing and chest pain, always searching for any signs of an impending heart attack. And, since a tendency of health-anxious people is to engage in all-or-nothing thinking, any time Erick did notice a bodily sensation, he'd automatically place himself in the dangerously ill or 'heart attack' category.

Now, it's not to say that Erick's concerns about heart health aren't valid. Obviously, we have all been told that heart disease is one of the leading causes of death. But does it mean that having one or two risk factors will inevitably result in death by heart attack? No. If he maintains a healthy lifestyle, participates in the appropriate screenings and tests as well as follows his doctors' recommendations, he can significantly reduce risk. Further, even if Erick develops some form of heart disease, it does not automatically mean he will have a heart attack.

If I suspect that a client holds rigid views about health and is assuming any diagnosis is likely to be the worst-case scenario, we will often collaboratively explore the variety of possible medical conditions that lie in the middle of the spectrum. One way to focus less on the worst-case scenario is to build the habit of considering the vast majority of medical conditions that are treatable and able to be managed or overcome.

Erick and I discussed how many cardiovascular health issues, such as hypertension, arrhythmia, coronary heart disease and heart murmur, can be effectively managed with lifestyle changes, medications, surgeries and device implantation as necessary. Erick is also fortunate his health insurance coverage gives him access to comprehensive disease management programs. We also explored the variety of ways he would be able to emotionally cope with these medical conditions if he were to get diagnosed. This included his faith, support from his wife, friends, relatives and broader social network, running half marathons and his passion for his career. Overall, Erick was able to see that there were more than just two options of being in good health or getting sick and dying.

Practice seeing health in a new way

Spend some time in the middle of the spectrum. Think of a time recently that you were viewing health as dichotomous. Perhaps you were catastrophizing about a symptom you had. Build the habit of considering other diagnoses that are curable or manageable. List them out. Then write out the available treatment options and how you would cope, physically and emotionally.

If necessary, you may use the internet to help you come up with responses in terms of how you would cope or treat it. However, use your discretion about doing this. If you think this will be too difficult for you to do without looking up other, unhelpful information, then take precautions. Ask a loved one to complete that part of this exercise. They can provide the information to you and you can write it down here.

Lethal or terminal	**Middle of the health spectrum**	**Perfect health**
	Diagnosis and coping	

Challenge assumptions by learning from others

Earlier in the chapter, I discussed my experiences working as a mental health clinician in a hospital. I interacted with many patients who had moderate to serious medical conditions, many of whom were receiving effective treatments and coping well. This helped me to recognize the power of human resilience, emotionally and physically. Talking to and learning from people who are managing serious medical issues can help you reshape your assumption that disease is an automatic death sentence.

It is time to gain a fresh perspective on this. One way to do this is to conduct interviews with people who have suffered with an illness or who are currently suffering with an illness. One of my clients, Shay, feared getting an illness because she feared it would kill her, first and foremost. However, she also made other assumptions about what it would be like to live with a serious disease. She assumed she would inevitably be unable to care for herself, humiliated, isolated, rejected by loved ones and in continuous, excruciating pain.

Now, it isn't to say that Shay's fears aren't real challenges faced by people with serious diseases. However, Shay was assuming the worst-case scenario in all of these categories. She not only assumed that she would face every one of these challenges, but she also assumed she would not be able to cope and would, consequently, live in utter despair. We developed a plan for her to interview five people who had either: (1) faced a serious illness in the past; and/or (2) were currently facing a serious illness.

Shay interviewed people in her social circles, including a combination of acquaintances, colleagues and close loved ones. Although learning about people's experiences with a variety of diseases was challenging, overall she gained a lot from this activity. Of course, people shared their struggles but she was also able to witness people's strength, resilience and hope, despite what they had been through. In fact, one person shared with Shay about how much their disease helped them turn their life around in a positive way.

Try this exercise. Start by thinking of three to five people you could interview that have faced a medical condition, currently or in the past. The goal of this exercise is not to focus on the threat of disease and sickness. Yes, you will learn about their experiences with disease, obviously. But the goal is to learn about how they were able to *cope* with their disease. So keep that in mind throughout this process. If you spend most of your time focusing on the symptoms and diagnosis, it might end up being counterproductive.

When you are inviting people to interview, explain that you are hoping to learn about how people are able to cope with illness. Many people appreciate being able to share their stories! Below are a few suggestions for interview questions. Of course, feel free to include any additional questions that might help you gain more insight into their experiences with coping.

Table 1 Potential interview questions

Support from loved ones	Did you have support from loved ones? Who? How did they support you or make you feel safer? How were they there for you (e.g. emotional or psychological support, intellectual support with help understanding the disease or having to navigate through medical decisions or the details around caring for oneself, physical assistance with daily tasks or getting to the doctor, financial assistance)?
Emotional support from professionals or peers going through something similar	Did you participate in individual or group counseling of any kind? If so, was it beneficial? How so? Did you have any support from peers who have been through something similar or who are supporting someone who has been through something similar? Where did you meet these individuals (online or in-person support group, interaction at medical facilities, at church or community center, in an online community support group like a Facebook Group or something else)? How did this help?
Experiences with treatment and doctors or other medical professionals	How were your experiences with getting treatment for this disease? Was the treatment helpful/ beneficial/effective? As you faced hardships in your treatment or healing process, how were you able to cope with these challenges? Did you have any positive experiences with your doctors, nurses or other medical professionals throughout your treatment? Can you describe these experiences and how they helped you?
Personal resilience and perspective	Did you acquire new skills or learn anything throughout the process of managing this disease? Did you surprise yourself in your ability to cope with this disease? In what way are you a different person today than you were when you first got diagnosed? Do you have any new insight from these experiences? How has it reshaped your perspective on life, yourself, your priorities or your loved ones? How are you different?

A few reflection questions to consider after the interviews

1 What were some of the key takeaway messages about coping?

2 Did you learn anything about coping that surprised you? Did you learn anything that inspired you or helped put things into perspective?

3 Was there anything that resonated with you in particular (e.g. a coping strategy that stood out to you or a specific outlook that you think might be helpful for you)?
4 How can you integrate what you learned about coping into your views about your own ability to cope with disease?
5 Relating back to you- how might you be able to cope with a medical condition (whether in the future or a current medical condition)? What strengths do you have that would help you cope? What resources do you have (e.g. socially, spiritually, emotionally, financially, medically, psychologically)?

Challenging beliefs about being weak and vulnerable

A key reason health-anxious people overestimate the severity of getting a disease is because they assume they are weak and unable to cope with disease. It can be helpful to explore this belief and evaluate the validity of their presumed vulnerability. As we did in Chapter 3 (see this activity to refresh your memory on all the details), we can use a core belief exercise to critically analyze these assumptions. This process allows you to identify and evaluate each piece of 'evidence' for your belief. The goal is to learn to recognize your own physical strength, resilience and capability for coping with, treating or overcoming the vast majority of illnesses and diseases. Notably, if you have a medical condition, you can also challenge any beliefs you hold about not being able to cope with the disease.

Now, in some cases, people are actually dealing with serious or debilitating diseases and have compromised immune systems. In those particular cases, of course, they may be particularly vulnerable to illness and the appropriate steps need to be taken to protect their health, as advised by their doctors.

That said, many people who live with this assumption are not weak or vulnerable to disease to the extent they are assuming. This leads them to live in fear of all diseases because they rationalize that any symptom could be the beginning of the end. Even if you have a medical condition, you may be underestimating your own strength and ability to cope with your condition. You can challenge these beliefs just like I did with Sadie in the example below.

Sadie

My client, Sadie, had a few minor health problems that she was managing with medication and diet, including irritable bowel syndrome and other gastrointestinal issues as well as high cholesterol. Even though she was young and in overall decent health, she had an ongoing intense fear of being diagnosed with a serious disease. She did not believe she had the physical strength or resilience to put up a good fight and, thus, remained convinced that many diseases would result in her debilitation and/or death. Her assumption about her inability to cope with disease only further reinforced her fear of it. Thus, any symptom or 'sign' of disease was especially scary for her, since she believed getting a disease meant she would not survive. Below is the core belief exercise I did with Sadie.

Steps to modify core beliefs

Step 1: We write the maladaptive core belief at the top of the worksheet. In this case, *I am weak and, therefore, likely to be killed by most diseases.*

Step 2: We then come up with a new, more adaptive belief. In this case, *I am generally pretty healthy and would be able to cope with, manage and/or overcome most diseases.*

Step 3: We assess the degree to which you believe both beliefs (0–100, with 100 being the strongest). Remember that core beliefs are not permanent or static. They fluctuate depending on a variety of factors and can also change over time. This helps to highlight that important point.

Step 4: We make two lists, one to gather evidence for the old core belief and one to gather evidence for the new core belief.

Step 5: We begin collecting evidence for the old, maladaptive core belief.

Step 6: After we have finished, we go through the evidence and look for any potential thinking errors or inaccuracies. We write out the reframes next to each piece of evidence.

Step 7: We then list out all the evidence that contradicts the old core belief and appears to support the new core belief.

Step 8: We look through all of the evidence on both sides and then assess the extent to which you believe the old core belief as well as the extent to which you believe the new one. Please note that if you believe the new core belief even a tad more (and the old core belief a little less),

I would conclude the intervention was helpful. Even a ten-point difference can improve your daily experiences to some extent.

Step 9: After you complete the exercise, continue collecting evidence on an ongoing basis.

Additional tips for core belief worksheets

1 When you are identifying evidence for the old, maladaptive core belief, make sure you are including everything, even if you know the piece of evidence is silly.
2 Make sure you document the extent to which you believe both beliefs, before and after the intervention.
3 You will not change your beliefs entirely during this one activity, so use this worksheet as a starting point.

Old core belief

I AM WEAK AND, THEREFORE, LIKELY TO BE KILLED BY MOST DISEASES.

How much do you believe this core belief (*before the intervention*)? (0–100) **70**

EVIDENCE THAT SEEMS TO SUPPORT THE OLD CORE BELIEF (WITH REFRAME)

- I am overweight and that can lead to many health problems, making me more vulnerable if I did get diagnosed with something. *REFRAME: Yes, being overweight can contribute to health problems. However, I am only slightly overweight, and I still live a relatively healthy lifestyle. I don't smoke, don't do drugs, don't drink that much, eat relatively healthy and walk regularly. These things all help keep my body strong.*
- My dad died fairly young and, therefore, I am likely to die young too. *REFRAME: My dad is not the same person as me and genetics are not deterministic. Also, my dad was obese and had multiple health issues that he did not manage responsibly for many years before he died. He often did not listen to his doctors, forgot to take or refill his medications and did not take good care of his body. Lifestyle played a big role in his health issues.*

- I hear random stories sometimes about healthy people who get diagnosed with something and are dead months or even weeks later. It makes it seem hopeless, like if you get a disease, there is not much you can do and you are eventually going to die from it. *REFRAME: I didn't actually know the people in most of the stories I have heard about someone who gets a diagnosis and rapidly declines/dies. I know a lot more people, personally, who have been diagnosed with different things and have all been either cured or able to live with it and keep it under control.*

New core belief

I AM GENERALLY PRETTY HEALTHY AND WOULD BE ABLE TO COPE WITH, MANAGE AND/OR OVERCOME MOST DISEASES.

How much do you believe this core belief (*before the intervention*)? (0–100) **15**

EVIDENCE THAT CONTRADICTS THE OLD CORE BELIEF AND SUPPORTS THE NEW ONE

- I have a few minor health problems and they have been pretty easy to manage and keep under control by medication and taking better care of myself. My gastroenterologist and primary care physician have done a good job at addressing issues as they have come up. It gives me confidence that I would have the resources to cope with more difficult issues, if necessary.
- I am only 30, and being young could make me even more likely to be able to beat or manage a disease.
- I follow all screening recommendations by doctors/experts (e.g. mammograms, monthly breast exams, routine blood work, dental cleanings, eye exams) so if I do get a serious disease, I am likely to catch something early, which makes it more treatable.
- I exercise regularly and can do most physically demanding activities. I am also able to exercise for extended periods of time. More recently, I have even started lifting weights and doing more intensive cardio. I am sure this strengthens my body and increases my ability to cope with disease better if I were to get something.
- Every time I have gotten sick, I've recovered in the average amount of time either without medicine or with standard treatment.

- I have seen many people in my personal life (many older or less healthy than me) survive and even thrive despite having serious diseases (e.g. colon cancer, breast cancer, type 1 diabetes, autoimmune diseases, brain tumor).
- The survival rates for cancer and other serious diseases are extremely promising and continue to get better as more treatments become available, so there are a lot of medical treatments/resources that would support my ability to overcome it even if I did get a disease.

How much do you believe this core belief (*after the intervention*)? (0–100) **75**

In this chapter, you learned that people with health anxiety tend to overestimate the severity of disease. Why do we do this? For one, we tend to assume we are weak and vulnerable, making us unable to cope with disease. We also tend to hold rigid health beliefs, assuming that one is either very healthy or very sick, with little room for anything in between those two extremes. However, remember that you are not stuck with these thought patterns. All thoughts and beliefs are malleable.

Continue the work. Identify thinking errors and practice your new Socratic dialogue skills. Be intentional about paying attention to the many stories around you of people facing medical conditions and still thriving with less-than-perfect health. Learn to live in the middle of the spectrum. And last but certainly not least, acknowledge and embrace your own strength and resilience, both physically and emotionally. You can improve all of this by working on it a little each day.

References

1 Boersma P, Black LI, Ward BW. Prevalence of multiple chronic conditions among US adults, 2018. *Preventing Chronic Disease.* 2020;17(17). <https://doi.org/10.5888/pcd17.200130>

2 Hacker K. The burden of chronic disease. *Mayo Clinic Proceedings: Innovations, Quality & Outcomes.* 2024;8(1):112–119. <https://doi.org/10.1016/j.mayocpiqo.2023.08.005>

3 Mahara G, Tian C, Xu X, Wang W. Revolutionising health care: Exploring the latest advances in medical sciences. *Journal of Global Health.* 2023;13(13):03042. <https://doi.org/10.7189/jogh.13.03042>

4 Mishra S. Does modern medicine increase life-expectancy: Quest for the Moon Rabbit? *Indian Heart Journal.* 2016 Jan–Feb;68(1):19–27. <10.1016/j.ihj.2016.01.003. Epub 2016 Jan 18. PMID: 26896262; PMCID: PMC4759485.>

5 Centers for Disease Control and Prevention. Life expectancy. Centers for Disease Control and Prevention. Published February 7, 2023. <https://www.cdc.gov/nchs/fastats/life-expectancy.htm>

6 Crimmins EM. Lifespan and Healthspan: Past, present, and promise. *The Gerontologist.* 2015;55(6):901–911. <https://doi.org/10.1093/geront/gnv130>

7 American Cancer Society. Survival rates for breast cancer. www.cancer.org. Published March 1, 2023. <https://www.cancer.org/cancer/types/breast-cancer/understanding-a-breast-cancer-diagnosis/breast-cancer-survival-rates.html>

5

Live more comfortably with bodily sensations and symptoms

People with health anxiety incorrectly assume all bodily sensations and symptoms are due to an underlying medical condition. They tend to notice a change in their bodies and jump to conclusions about the potential diseases that could be the cause, or they jump to conclusions about the symptom pointing to an imminent medical crisis. This is why you may search for immediate answers as soon as any symptom or bodily sensation emerges. However, many physiological sensations are just part of normal, self-regulatory biological processes and responses to your environment. The more that you can learn to accept that being symptom-free is an unnecessary and unattainable goal, the less distressed you will become when you experience new symptoms or bodily sensations.

My client, Sandy, became overwhelmed with anxiety whenever she noticed heart palpitations or an increased heart rate. Despite multiple tests with no concerning results, Sandy remained convinced changes in her heart rate meant her heart was struggling to function properly. She worried that if she ignored this concerning symptom, she would have a stroke or heart attack. Thus, she refrained from exercise or any activity that could increase her heart rate to 'dangerous' levels. She also made sure she always remained near medical facilities so that she could frequently visit urgent care or the emergency room to confirm these symptoms weren't a sign of an impending stroke or heart attack.

Sandy mistakenly believed that any change in heart rate must be from an underlying medical problem rather than recognizing that this symptom could be due to normal, benign biological and environmental factors. She also engaged in body vigilance and paid selective attention to her heart rate, including checking her BPM multiple times throughout the day. This made her much more likely to notice any bodily sensations, including minor changes and/or changes due to normal, random body noise. Of course, she was then more likely to experience a greater increase in anxiety symptoms, which only further exacerbated these types of symptoms.

People with health anxiety also tend to assume that the physiological symptoms that accompany anxiety are harmful or dangerous. This is known as 'anxiety sensitivity' or 'distress intolerance.' They might detect some kind of a threat (e.g. a new symptom, news about someone's health, another type of threat unrelated to disease) and begin to feel anxious arousal. The physiological symptoms associated with anxious arousal are then misinterpreted as being due to a serious medical problem or a sign of an impending medical emergency. They might fear they will spiral out of control and 'go crazy' or that their body will not be able to withstand the pressure if the anxiety symptoms become too intense. I often say that panic attacks and health anxiety are 'besties' because both involve a fear of and focus on bodily sensations and symptoms.

The human body makes noise

Our bodies make 'noise' for a variety of reasons that are not always identifiable or due to a medical crisis or serious disease. On a daily basis, we experience bodily sensations from normal, self-regulatory biological processes, changes in routines such as sleep, diet or exercise, emotional and physiological reactions to our environment as well as benign or minor medical conditions. For example, self-regulatory biological processes can lead to digestive noises, joint sounds, heart and blood flow sounds, respiratory noises, peristaltic sounds, muscle contractions, eustachian tube sounds and nervous system noises.[1,2,3,4]

The mind–body connection is one example of how our bodies can make 'noise' that is not indicative of a threat (i.e. disease or urgent medical crisis). Our minds and physical bodies are inherently interconnected in a complex, bidirectional relationship.[5] When we have certain thoughts and experience emotions (e.g. anger, sadness, stress, anxiety, excitement), these experiences produce physiological sensations. Further, our physiological state also impacts our mental state. For instance, when one exercises, this releases certain chemicals, which can evoke emotional experiences of happiness and positivity.

When facing a stressful or anxiety-provoking situation, our brains release stress hormones, which cause a wide variety of physiological sensations (e.g. increased heart rate, change in breathing patterns, increased muscle tension, burst of energy). When in danger, this is an adaptive response to protect us by preparing us to fight or flee. Of course, the body can produce a stress reaction to situations that are non-threatening as well, which happens often with clinical anxiety. These symptoms are often misinterpreted by a health-anxious person as being indicative of a health problem. Which of these symptoms tend to trigger the most anxiety for you?

As mentioned in Chapter 2, people with health anxiety tend to engage in 'body vigilance,' in which they pay selective attention to every bodily sensation and symptom. This creates a heightened awareness of every sound the body makes, even the natural sounds

Table 1 Common symptoms associated with the fight–flight–freeze response

Rapid and shallow breathing or breathlessness	Rapid heart beat and increase in blood pressure	Sweating	Dilated pupils	Blurred vision
Pain or tightness in chest	Seeing spots or light sensitivity	Muscle tension	Muscle twitching	Eye blinking
Trembling or shaking	Joint pain	Headaches	Nausea, bloating, consti-pation, diarrhea	Decrease in salivation or dry mouth
Lightheadedness and dizziness	Confusion and difficulty concentrating	Feelings of unreality/ dream state	Loss of energy or drained feeling	Pale or flushed skin
Feeling keyed up or on edge	Restlessness	Clammy skin, cold to the touch	Increased alertness and sharpened senses	Losing control of bladder or bowels
Throat tight-ening sensation or difficulty swallowing	Disrupted sleep patterns	Suppressed hunger	Digestive issues	Irritability

from normal biological processes. In addition, a health-anxious person is more likely to experience physiological symptoms of anxiety. All of this leads one to notice more symptoms or sensations and then to interpret them as signs of a medical crisis or serious disease. Not surprisingly, an important part of improving health anxiety is to help one to learn how to refrain from engaging in body vigilance. Later in this chapter, you will learn techniques to accomplish this.

Misinterpretations of bodily sensations and symptoms

When we believe most or all bodily sensations and symptoms are dangerous (i.e. indicative of medical emergency or serious disease), we misinterpret these sensations and symptoms. Recall that core beliefs are the lens through which we see the world and, as such, guide how we interpret the situations we face in our daily lives. As illustrated in the diagram below, if you believe that anxiety is dangerous and/or that you must be symptom-free to be healthy, then you would naturally jump to conclusions or catastrophize whenever you notice a new bodily sensation.

It is tempting for a health-anxious person to assume they are simply more 'in tune' with their body and, therefore, more accurate in their judgments about symptoms. However, research shows the opposite: health anxiety is associated with biased and inaccurate interpretations of bodily sensations and symptoms.[6] The more one changes these beliefs and begins to understand the normalcy of body noise and the mind–body connection, the less likely one will be to assume that all bodily sensations are dangerous or indicative of disease.

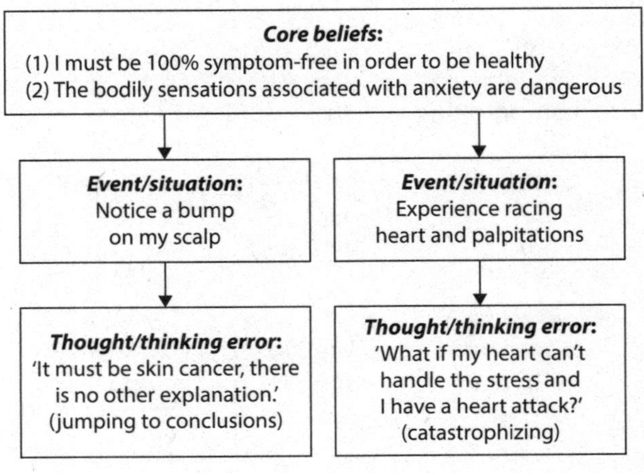

Core beliefs:
(1) I must be 100% symptom-free in order to be healthy
(2) The bodily sensations associated with anxiety are dangerous
Event/situation:
Notice a bump on my scalp
Event/situation:
Experience racing heart and palpitations
Thought/thinking error:
'It must be skin cancer, there is no other explanation.' (jumping to conclusions)
Thought/thinking error:
'What if my heart can't handle the stress and I have a heart attack?' (catastrophizing)

Beliefs about the danger of bodily sensations and thinking errors

Of course, because we assume that bodily sensations and symptoms are a sign of danger, we are inclined to misinterpret the meaning of our sensations and symptoms, resulting in all sorts of thinking errors. For example, if you believe that bodily sensations, even those caused by anxiety, have the potential to spiral out of control and become lethal, you would then assume you are in great danger when a new sensation emerges. Or if you believe you must be 100 percent symptom-free to be healthy, then any new symptom would mean you are *not* healthy and, thus, should be of grave concern. Below are a few examples of the thinking errors my clients and I have engaged in due to underlying beliefs about the danger of bodily sensations and symptoms.

> All-or-nothing thinking: Viewing health and bodily sensations and symptoms in only two categories. One is either healthy, with an absence of bodily sensations and 'safe,' or ill, with the presence of bodily sensations and 'in great danger.'

My client, Todd, feared having a heart attack and he developed a terrible habit of vigilantly watching for any 'signs.' Over time, this preoccupation and growing fear led him to see his heart health as dichotomous. If he had no symptoms or bodily sensations, his heart was healthy and he was 'safe.' However, if any bodily sensations emerged that he believed could be linked to his heart (e.g. increased BPM, tingling sensation in arms, pain in chest), it automatically meant he had poor heart function, would eventually have a heart attack and was, thus, 'in great danger.' In reality, one's heart rate might increase for a variety of non-threatening reasons (e.g. changes in diet or sleep patterns, random body noise, anxiety, exercise, certain medications). As Todd's anxiety grew, he tried to control his heart rate by avoiding any activity that might increase it.

> Anxiety intolerance: Assuming that the anxiety or discomfort will last indefinitely or will cause one to lose control or experience harmful medical or physical consequences.

Health-anxious people commonly assume the physiological symptoms produced by anxiety could be dangerous. One of my biggest triggers has always been shortness of breath. For a long time, whenever I experienced breathlessness, even if the cause was fairly obvious (e.g.

being anxious or walking up a flight of stairs), I would start spiraling, convinced that the anxiety symptom itself was dangerous and I was about to suffocate. Even though I recognized it was only anxiety, I worried that my body would somehow collapse or break down under the pressure of the anxiety symptoms. What if my lungs just couldn't get enough air and the anxiety itself caused me to suffocate?

The fear of the immediate medical consequences of anxiety is a common concern among those who experience panic attacks. Lucky for me, I had a history of panic attacks and health anxiety. Thus, I lived in fear of *both* the immediate and eventual medical consequences of anxiety. In reality, anxiety symptoms, while extremely uncomfortable, are not dangerous in any way. Our bodies produce physiological symptoms when we are anxious to protect us from harm, not put us in danger.

Catastrophizing: Predicting only the most disastrous outcomes when it comes to your health. Any unexplained bodily sensation or symptom is a sign of disease or medical emergency, any of which would presumably result in the worst-case scenario.

One of my clients, Angie, often experienced dizziness when she was in an anxious state. Even though she recognized, most of the time, the dizziness was due to anxiety and not an underlying disease, she was convinced that the anxiety symptoms would lead to catastrophic outcomes. She believed the dizziness would lead her to faint, hit her head and subsequently die after hitting her head on the floor. As this fear grew, Angie would even grip furniture or the walls as she walked to the bathroom, 'just in case' she had a random dizzy spell, to keep her from falling to her death.

Reconsider view of bodily sensations and symptoms

One way to improve health anxiety is to evaluate and reconsider assumptions and develop more adaptive beliefs about bodily sensations and symptoms. Specifically, I want you to see that you do not need to be 100 percent symptom-free at all times to be unhealthy, which is both an unnecessary and unattainable goal. I also want you to understand that not every symptom or bodily sensation has an identifiable medical explanation or is due to some kind of medical emergency or serious disease. Several cognitive and behavioral techniques can help you to reshape how you see bodily sensations.

Socratic dialogue

Socratic dialogue is a foundational skill taught in CBT to challenge thinking errors. Of course, in this chapter we will challenge thoughts related to the danger of bodily sensations and symptoms. If it helps, review the section in Chapter 3 on why and how using Socratic dialogue can help you reshape biases and distorted thinking. In short, use the questions below as inspiration to help you critically analyze your thoughts and seek out any potential inconsistencies, contradictions or exceptions. The goal is to help you learn to view bodily sensations and symptoms in a more balanced way.

Table 2 Examples of Socratic questions related to the danger of bodily sensations

What thoughts ran through my mind when I first noticed this symptom or these symptoms? Could these thoughts be intensifying the symptoms?

- Is it possible that these bodily sensations could be due to benign bodily fluctuations or the fight-or-flight response? Could I commit to learning more about the science behind random body noise?
- Could I learn to practice mindfulness and acceptance of random bodily sensations without judgment of them?
- What are my normal physiological responses to anxiety (i.e. my specific patterns)? Is it possible that my current bodily sensation or symptom is a part of my normal pattern of response to an anxiety trigger?
- Did something happen recently that made me more anxious and, thus, could have brought on these symptoms (e.g. hearing a scary health story, having a new health concern, noticing a change in my body)?
- Could there be other, harmless or benign explanations for these symptoms such as caffeine intake, change in diet, lack of sleep or stress?
- Have I been concerned about these bodily sensations in the past? How often did they turn out to be something normal, minor or benign? How can I draw from these experiences to challenge any anxious thoughts?
- Have I discussed these bodily sensations with a healthcare professional (recently or in the past)? What were their professional opinions, diagnoses, recommendations?
- Have I ever been harmed from anxiety? Has it ever been permanent or does it always dissipate? If I've ruled out any major health concerns related to these symptoms, why does this concern continue? Is it possible that I am seeking certainty about my health? If so, can I consider why this is an impossible and unnecessary goal?

Table 2 (*Continued*)

• Is it possible that I am jumping to conclusions or catastrophizing about the danger of these bodily sensations (whether an immediate or eventual medical catastrophe)? How so? • Can I walk myself through specifically *how* these symptoms could be life-threatening? For instance, if I am afraid that experiencing 'too much' anxiety will lead to a heart attack, how exactly would this happen? Is it possible that my theory goes against what we know about human physiology? • Am I allowing my imagination to run wild about the symptom and then stopping at the feared event? Could it be helpful to walk through the entire scenario? For instance, if I fear fainting, instead of stopping at the point in the story in which I faint, could I walk through the rest of the story? If I fainted at the store, for instance, could I imagine myself fainting for a few seconds and then returning to consciousness, other customers helping me stand up, calling a loved one to come get me and going home or to the doctor? • Do I think it is possible that by hyper focusing on my bodily sensations, I am increasing anxiety (and bringing on even more sensations) as well as making myself more likely to notice every sensation and symptom? • What would I say to a friend if they experienced this symptom and thought they were about to have an immediate or eventual medical crisis? • How is my fear of symptoms and bodily sensations impacting my life? How could life be different if I learned to accept bodily sensations as normal and not scary? What could be the benefits of changing this way of thinking?

Practice makes perfect

Let's continue exercising these skills with practice. Review the list of common thinking errors, and, for the next week, document your thoughts in a thought record. Any time you think you might be assuming that a bodily sensation/symptom is dangerous or indicative of a serious health concern, practice identifying your related thinking errors. Next, challenge those thinking errors with the relevant Socratic questions above. I also challenge you to practice coming up with your own questions as you see fit.

Common thinking errors

- All-or-nothing thinking
- Jumping to conclusions
- Catastrophizing
- Emotional reasoning
- Mental filter/Tunnel vision

- Unrealistic expectations
- Overgeneralization
- Magical thinking

Thought record to identify thinking errors and challenge thoughts

Date & situation or trigger & level of anxiety (1–10)

January 10

Noticed a random heart palpitation that seemed to come out of nowhere.

Anxiety: 8/10

Automatic thought about the situation & level of concern (1–10)

Why would my heart suddenly beat rapidly for no reason? This is not normal. I know my test results came back fine but maybe this is a new issue. I've always felt that a heart attack would be what kills me. I don't think I should work out today after all, just in case there actually is something wrong with my heart. I don't want to put too much pressure on it and risk having a heart attack.

Level of concern: 9/10

Potential thinking errors

(1) Mental filter/Tunnel vision: focusing on certain information that supports my assumption that I am likely to have a heart attack (experiencing a heart palpitation), while ignoring other information (normal test results).

(2) Emotional reasoning: believing I am likely to die from a heart attack because it feels true, even with a lack of evidence (normal test results).

(3) Jumping to conclusions: making assumptions about one's overall health based on little evidence (one time noticing a heart palpitation).

(4) Catastrophizing: assuming that even if there is an issue with my heart, it automatically means heart attack and death.

Response to thoughts or challenging with Socratic dialogue

I am jumping to conclusions and catastrophizing about a fairly normal bodily sensation (heart palpitations). Heart palpitations can be normal. They can also be a common anxiety symptom. My doctors have recently ruled out any major concerns with my heart based on tests. It is highly unlikely that my cardiovascular health has changed dramatically since the tests were done a few months ago. Also, I always feel like something is wrong because I overestimate my chances of having a serious disease or medical emergency. Thus, my feelings aren't a reliable indicator. I am always on the lookout for evidence that I will have a heart attack.

Date & situation or trigger & level of anxiety (1–10)

January 15

I was running at the gym and felt hot and out of breath. I suddenly started to feel anxious about the fact that it was hot and I couldn't breathe. And then I started to worry that if the anxiety got worse, I wouldn't be able to catch my breath and would suffocate.

Anxiety: 9/10

Automatic thought about the situation & level of concern (1–10)

What if I am an odd case of someone with undiagnosed asthma or lung disease? My cousin got diagnosed with asthma as an adult. And then what if my anxiety spins out of control, making it difficult to breathe and then I suffocate because I had an underlying issue that I didn't even know about? Or even if I don't have a lung issue, what if I die simply because my body can't handle all of this anxiety and I am unable to catch my breath? Maybe I should leave and go to urgent care on the way home just to be sure this doesn't happen.

Level of concern: 9/10

Potential thinking errors

(1) Catastrophizing: predicting the most unlikely disastrous outcomes: that I would not only have an undiagnosed medical condition but that this condition would cause me to suddenly die.

(2) All-or-nothing thinking: assuming that, even if I were to have a lung issue, it would automatically result in death.

(3) Overgeneralization: making broad conclusions based on one health-related event (i.e. I have undiagnosed asthma because my cousin got diagnosed as an adult).

Response to thoughts or challenging with Socratic dialogue

I am catastrophizing and assuming two worst-case scenarios will happen at once. I am assuming that (a) I would have an undiagnosed lung issue; and (b) my anxiety symptoms will kill me because of an undiagnosed lung issue. In reality, I most likely do not have an undiagnosed lung issue out of nowhere, with no symptoms. Even if I did, it does not mean I will die from anxiety symptoms. I am also overgeneralizing—my cousin had many symptoms prior to being diagnosed and went to the doctor with these concerns. I have no other symptoms of a lung issue (other than feeling anxious). Lastly, having asthma does not mean dying—it is a minor health issue that can be controlled.

The 'Examine the Evidence' exercise

My client, Maya, believed she was prone to heart disease and feared having a heart attack. Even though medical evaluations and test results determined her cardiovascular health to be fine, she remained convinced she had an undiagnosed heart condition. As a result, she feared any bodily sensations she thought might be a sign of a heart issue. She became especially nervous any time her heart rate increased because she worried that her 'weak heart' would easily become overwhelmed if she pushed it beyond its limits through stress, anxiety or any kind of physical exertion. She refrained from exercising, having sex, drinking coffee and even walking up a flight of stairs. We decided to examine the evidence for her anxious thoughts about the danger of her bodily sensations.

Tips for completing the exercise

Recall from Chapter 3 this strategy is used to critically evaluate potentially distorted thoughts. Remember, we genuinely want to better understand the evidence behind your thoughts, as we are not aiming to think more positively but to think more logically. Now, I will show you how Maya and I documented the evidence for her anxious thoughts. Below are a few tips for completing this exercise.

- Open up a google doc or piece of paper and create two lists: evidence *for* the thought and evidence *against* the thought.
- Identify the anxious thought and write it down. Be as specific as possible.
- Assess the extent to which you believe this thought (on a scale of 0–100).
- Collect the evidence *for* your anxious thought.
- Collect the evidence *against* the thought.
- Return to the evidence *for* the thought section and reframe or challenge any 'evidence' that seems biased or inaccurate.
- Note: because your anxiety may be leading you to believe something is 'evidence' when it isn't, you need to give yourself the opportunity to challenge it. It can be helpful to write or type the reframes in a different color (I prefer red). This helps you to recognize the distinction between the evidence *for* the anxious thought and your reframes or arguments *against* any biases in your evidence for the anxious thought. I find making this distinction particularly useful when we go back to review all of the data together.
- Review all the evidence together and reassess the extent to which you believe your distressing thought. This allows us to see whether the exercise was helpful at all. It doesn't need to be drastic. Even a reduction by ten points might make you feel less anxious.
- Identify a few alternative explanations for the symptom.

Examine the Evidence

Anxious thought: My heart may not be able to withstand the pressure if the anxiety becomes too overwhelming (or if I put too much strain on my heart through physical exertion), and I could, consequently, have a heart attack.

Degree of belief before the exercise (0–100): **85/100**

Degree of belief after the exercise (0–100): **50/100**

Evidence FOR the thought

- Sometimes my heart races so fast that it seems like I am about to have a heart attack, such as when I am anxious or when I work out or engage in physical activity. *REFRAME: Feelings are not facts. I often have a 'sneaky feeling' that something is seriously wrong with my body and I am almost always wrong. My anxiety makes me more likely to jump to conclusions and think something is wrong, even when there is more reason to think a racing heart isn't a big deal.*

- My maternal grandfather had a sudden, massive heart attack when he was 58 and died so heart disease is in my family. *REFRAME: Although genetics can put me at a higher risk for heart disease, I have had many tests done to check my overall cardiovascular health and so far there have been no concerns. Also, one family member's health situation does not automatically determine my own health situation. And even if I did inherit a health condition, it doesn't mean I'd have a heart attack and die—I'd probably be able to manage it with lifestyle changes and medication or other treatments.*
- When my anxiety is high, I have also noticed other symptoms that seem similar to symptoms people have when they have a heart attack (tightness in chest, shortness of breath). *REFRAME: Yes, these are all symptoms of a heart attack but they are also symptoms of anxiety. My doctor (and therapist) have told me once we rule out any cardiovascular concerns (which we have), we can then assume the symptoms are due to anxiety, particularly when I am feeling anxious. In these cases, I have been super anxious.*
- Even though the doctors have run all the tests to make sure there are no issues with my heart, they could have missed something. *REFRAME: Anything is possible but it is unlikely that every doctor and every test missed something important. I can't be 100 percent sure that I won't have a heart attack but I also can't be sure that I won't get violently attacked by someone on the street. It's life.*

Evidence AGAINST the thought

- I have had multiple tests done on many different occasions and everything came back normal, with no concerns about my cardiovascular health. If my heart really was 'weak,' something would have shown up.

- Physicians, including during ER, urgent care and PCP visits, have repeatedly told me that my heart fluttering and pounding is due to anxiety and, thus, not dangerous.
- I have had clinical anxiety, including panic attacks, for many years and have never had a heart attack or been physically harmed by my anxiety. I also know lots of people with anxiety and don't know anyone who has been harmed by intense anxiety symptoms. According to my doctor, the only way anxiety or panic could trigger an event or medical issue is if I had an underlying condition, which I do not have.
- I used to work out all of the time, including high-intensity workouts and running half marathons. I even ran a marathon once. Never have any of these activities had a negative impact on my health in any way. In fact, I noticed significant improvement in my health, including my cholesterol levels, when I was working out more intensively on a regular basis.
- Although people can have heart attacks from too much physical exertion if they already have an existing heart condition, working out doesn't cause heart conditions. Everyone I know who works out regularly is in decent health and, to my knowledge, has never developed a heart condition. Some people I know have told me they have improved cholesterol levels and blood pressure by working out more regularly.
- Overall, the human body is strong, resilient and functions in a way that makes it unlikely or perhaps even impossible for a healthy person with no cardiovascular conditions, like myself, to suddenly have a heart attack simply due to an increased heart rate. If this were true, people everywhere would be dropping like flies.

As a final step, ask yourself, is there an alternative way of viewing the situation? What is a new potential conclusion after reviewing all the evidence for and against the anxious thought?

In this case, Maya had been convinced that her heart was weak, which made her prone to a heart attack if she pushed her heart past its 'limit.' We reconsidered her assumption that her heart was weak. Given all her test results, her heart was actually strong and capable. We also reshaped Maya's assumption that anxiety was dangerous into the more adaptive view that anxiety was our body's natural response to protect us from harm and not put us in danger. Further, we reframed Maya's assumption that physical exertion could incite a heart attack into the more accurate view that physical activity was not only safe but actually improves cardiovascular health.

Again, the 'Examine the Evidence' exercise allows you to pull back and take a 'helicopter view' of the situation. You want to pull out all of the information floating around in your head because you likely just assume the 'evidence' you have conjured up is valid. This gives you the chance to evaluate said evidence and challenge it if you identify any biases in your assumptions. It also allows you to practice identifying evidence for an alternative viewpoint. Doing this can help you see the situation in a more balanced, adaptive way.

The 'Twist and Finish Out the Image' technique

When we jump to conclusions and catastrophize about a symptom or bodily sensation, we often picture a terrible event and then we abruptly end the daydream at the worst point in the scenario. This can happen with fears of immediate medical crises, like suffocating, losing consciousness or having a heart attack. It also can happen with fears of eventual medical crises, like being diagnosed with a terrible disease. We want to redirect the impulse to automatically conjure up worst-case scenario imagery and, instead, build a habit of imagining a more realistic and positive conclusion to the daydream.[7]

My client, Jayden, feared fainting so much she would not go to the grocery store alone. She feared she would faint and, without a loved one present to prevent her from sustaining an injury or get her the necessary medical assistance in time, she would not survive. Jayden admitted that she hadn't really thought through the details. She had lived with this fear for so long that her mind automatically jumped from a fainting spell to serious medical consequences and/or death.

We redirected Jayden's tendency by having her, instead, mentally walk through the entire scenario and envision a new, more realistic ending to her story. She imagined herself shopping alone and placing fruits and vegetables in her cart. She starts to feel lightheaded and her field of vision grows increasingly black as she loses consciousness and collapses on the floor. A few shoppers see her go down and kneel beside her. After a few moments, Jayden regains consciousness and opens her eyes to a few friendly faces, asking her if she is okay. She can stand back up again and one of the helpers suggests she calls someone to come pick her up. Her husband comes and takes her to the emergency room. A physical examination and blood test reveals she fainted due to anemia and Jayden is, subsequently, put on a treatment regimen.

You can use this technique with any feared scenario, whether it involves an immediate (e.g. sudden heart attack or stroke) or eventual medical catastrophe (e.g. getting diagnosed with and dying from a serious disease). This won't be easy at first. You have grown accustomed to jumping from the situation (noticing a new symptom) to a catastrophic ending. This takes time to change. However, the more you start to think in new ways, the more you will retrain your brain to jump to new, more realistic and positive conclusions. If you keep practicing, your brain will begin to do this automatically, as it once did when coming up with catastrophic scenarios.

Let's give it a try! Think of a recent situation in which you experienced an internal or external trigger, imagined the worst-case scenario and then ended the scenario at that point. If you can't think of a recent situation, use any situation from the past. Write it out. Next, twist the story a bit to make it more realistic and positive and then finish out the image or scenario.

Table 3 Twist and Finish Out the Image

Situation/Trigger	What happened and how did it end?	How can you twist the narrative and finish out the story?

Survey experiment

When we have anxiety, we spend so much time in our head that our biased interpretations seem completely normal. It can help to explore new perspectives. I know, in my case, seeing others view and deal with bodily sensations and symptoms in a practical, unruffled manner has helped me to see how extreme my own reactions are by comparison.

I remember in 6th grade, one of my fingers started peeling. I spent lunch crying to my friend Frances about how I was certain I had leprosy. She turned her hand over and spread out her fingers. *'See, look at my hand. It is much worse than yours. And I don't think I have leprosy.'* I couldn't believe she could be so cavalier—her skin was peeling everywhere! But the more I thought about her reaction, the better I felt. I thought, *Well, if she can have a symptom that bad and still be sure she is fine, maybe I am fine too?* I was so used to my catastrophic interpretation of every symptom that hearing a friend's interpretation of the same symptom was refreshing.

My client, Albert, was especially triggered by any forgetfulness, inattention or difficulty concentrating. He had a big fear of neurodegenerative diseases as well as a fear of suddenly losing his mind or 'going crazy.' Any time these symptoms presented, he assumed the worst-case scenario and feared for his immediate safety (e.g. suddenly losing his mind) as well as his long-term safety (e.g. slow cognitive decline due to being in the beginning stages of Alzheimer's). To help Albert step back and consider other perspectives, we implemented a little survey experiment. He surveyed ten people to ask about their experiences with these symptoms.

Table 4 Albert's survey questions

Have you ever experienced forgetfulness, inattention and/or difficulty concentrating?	Yes	No
If so, were you worried about these symptoms?	Yes	No
How did you interpret these symptoms?		

Albert's survey revealed most people had experienced forgetfulness, inattention and difficulty concentrating and were not worried about these symptoms. Specifically, all ten people reported forgetfulness at some point (many of them even stated they had had these symptoms many times at various points in their life). Out of the ten, eight people reported not being particularly worried about these symptoms because there were many potential explanations that weren't a big deal, such as not sleeping well, being stressed and busy, having ADHD, feeling depressed and being mentally preoccupied at the time. The two people that reported being worried elaborated they weren't worried about anything serious, like a neurological disorder, but had been experiencing either heightened stress or depression at that time and were, thus, concerned about their general mental health/physical health.

Albert was able to see, firsthand, that many of his loved ones, acquaintances and colleagues had experienced these symptoms at various points in their lives. This helped normalize these symptoms as a common occurrence because of many benign or minor reasons. Of course, as you might have guessed, none of the people he surveyed were diagnosed with Alzheimer's or lost their mind.

This experiment also gave Albert the opportunity to see the distinction between his and others' reactions to the same symptoms. He observed how others seemed to be, for the most part, at ease in the midst of experiencing forgetfulness and inattention because they knew it was most likely due to a non-catastrophic reason. This allowed Albert to get out of his own head and see the symptoms from others' perspectives.

Now, it's your turn! Think of a symptom that is a common trigger for you. Next, design a little survey experiment. Again, this is an opportunity to see others' perspectives and interpretations of similar symptoms. You likely spend a lot of time in your head, cycling through the same old distorted thoughts. Over time, this makes those thoughts seem more and more normal. Time to get out of your head and spend some time exploring the thought processes of others.

Recognizing the impact of selective attention

When you are in the market for a new car and have a specific one in mind, you start seeing that car everywhere. Our minds only have the capacity to focus on a limited number of objects in our environment at a time. Thus, we selectively attend to what matters to us the most in order to preserve this mental resource.

People with anxiety pay selective attention to 'threatening' stimuli in the environment. Threatening stimuli have many faces, so to speak, depending on what you are anxious about. People with health anxiety pay selective attention to bodily sensations because they want to be sure to identify any potential threat of disease.[7,8] Researchers refer to the lack of attentional control as Cognitive Attentional Syndrome (CAS), which describes the phenomenon of inflexible, self-focused attention, rumination and worry, cognitive inefficiency and maladaptive coping mechanisms, all of which keep one hyper focused on the threat.[9,10] In the case of health anxiety, the threat is the bodily sensation.

When we give an excessive amount of attention to every little peep that comes out of our bodies, we are more likely to notice bodily sensations and symptoms, including normal benign body noise. Of course, since we are constantly on the lookout for 'threat' or signs of disease, we are also likely to misinterpret any noise as being dangerous, whether it is immediate medical danger (e.g. a massive heart attack) or eventual medical danger (e.g. early-stage Alzheimer's disease). The hyper focus on the body may explain why people with health anxiety tend to notice more 'symptoms' than people without health anxiety. For example, you may be able to recall a time when someone talked about a rash or lice and suddenly you began to notice an itching sensation. This has happened to me on several occasions! It can be helpful to recognize the relationship between *body-focused attention* and *greater awareness of bodily sensations* to help you refrain from jumping to conclusions and, instead, see bodily sensations in a more balanced way.

Internal versus external-attention exercise

Try a ten-minute exercise to help increase your awareness of the impact of self-focused attention. Focus on an area of your body that concerns you for five minutes and then divert your attention away from your body and toward the external environment for five minutes. This will allow you to explore whether there are any differences in the bodily sensations you notice between the periods of self-focused attention and environmental-focused attention.

First, briefly prepare for this exercise. Pick an area of your body that is a common source of concern. I've included a list of bodily areas that are common concerns for people who tend to see bodily sensations as threatening, such as those with a history of health anxiety and panic attacks. Next, select a simple or mundane task from the list below. This will be the task you will use to redirect your attention to the external environment. If you prefer to do another type of simple, mundane activity that is not listed here, by all means go for it! This list is just to make the task simple and convenient.

Table 5 Bodily areas of concern and mundane task ideas

Bodily area of concern	Simple/mundane task or activity
• Head and brain • Neck and throat • Heart and cardiovascular system • Breathing and respiratory system • Abdomen and digestive system • Limbs and muscles • Skin and dermatological system • Reproductive system • Vision and eyes	• Doing the dishes • Vacuuming • Sweeping the floor • Folding the laundry • Gardening • Taking a walk • Eating a snack • Brushing your teeth • Washing your hands • Taking a shower

Five minutes of internal focus

For this portion of the activity, focus exclusively on the selected body area for five minutes, paying special attention to every sensation you notice.

General instructions

- Go to a quiet room or space where you will not be interrupted or distracted to remove yourself from any environmental distractions or noise.
- Sit or lie down in a comfortable position.
- Set a timer for five minutes and check your phone notifications are on silent.
- Close your eyes if you feel comfortable with this, as it can help minimize environmental distractions.
- For each bodily area you decide to focus on, follow the specific guidelines on what to pay attention to during this five-minute period.
- If at any point you notice your mind start to drift away from focusing on your bodily sensations, don't judge it. This is what our minds do. Simply redirect your attention back to the bodily area and continue.
- After the timer goes off, briefly jot down the sensations you notice.

Table 6 Specific guidelines for bodily areas

Body area	Guidelines
Head and scalp	Become more aware of the entire surface of your head and scalp. Notice every detail of your head and scalp, including the surface of your face, the skin across the surface of your head and hair follicles. Notice any sensations, including tension, warmth, coolness, tingling or itchiness. Intensify your focus on your head and scalp by moving your fingers across your face and through your hair or lightly massage your scalp to bring more attention to these sensations. Notice if there are any changes in sensations around your head and scalp during this period of deliberate focus.
Neck and throat	Focus your attention on the neck and throat area. Pay attention to the muscles in this area and the sensation of your breath passing through. Pay attention to the sensations as you swallow, scanning for any tightening of your throat muscles, the sounds you hear as you swallow, any sensation of a lump in your throat, scratchiness, dryness or tenderness. Bring even more attention to the sensations in your throat by clearing your throat, coughing or swallowing multiple times in a row. Notice any sensations in the neck area, such as tension or stiffness, warmth or coolness. Intensify the focus on your neck, becoming aware of the sensations in your neck as your breath passes through.
Heart and chest	Shift your attention to your heart area, around the center of your chest. Tune into any sensations you may feel in this area, such as a gentle or strong pulse or a warmth sensation. Notice the rhythm and pace of your heartbeat. Be present with these sensations. Notice when your heart changes rhythm. To intensify your focus and enhance awareness, you can place your hand on your chest.
Breathing and lungs	Begin by paying attention to your natural breath. Notice the sensation of your breath as you inhale and exhale. Feel the rise and fall of your breath or the expansion and contraction of your abdomen. Take a few minutes to explore your breath. Notice its temperature, texture and the movements associated with each breath. Be fully present with the process of breathing. Notice any variations in your breathing, such as shallow or deep breathing.

Table 6 (*Continued*)

Body area	Guidelines
Abdomen	Bring your attention to the abdomen area, noticing your stomach rise and fall as you breathe. Take a few moments to explore and take note of any sensations or sounds, such as rumbling or gurgling sounds, growling or grumbling, feeling full or bloated, any contraction or relaxation of stomach muscles, gas, cramps. Be fully present with the movements and sounds coming from your abdominal area. Pay attention to any shifts or variations in everything you observe.
Limbs and muscles	Focus your attention on your muscles and joints throughout your body, including all of your limbs. Start from the bottom of your neck and slowly work your way down your body, being sure to include your arms and legs as you work your way down. Choose a specific group of muscles, such as your biceps, thighs or shoulders. Notice any sounds or bodily sensations related to your muscles and joints. Scan the muscles throughout your body to become aware of any soreness, tenderness, tension, twitching or cramping. Also take note of any popping, clicking or cracking sounds from your joints, muscles and tendons.

Reflect on whether and how self-focused attention influenced your perception of bodily sensations. Are there any changes while you are deliberately focusing on these bodily sensations? Jot down all your thoughts right after this exercise.

Table 7 Thought record for experience with focusing on sensations

Bodily area of focus	**Observations during the focus period** What sensations did I notice? Were there any changes in intensity, duration or pattern of bodily sensations? Was I more aware of subtle movements in that bodily area during the exercise? What were my thoughts? Did my focus or thoughts seem to influence sensations?

Five minutes of external focus

After five minutes of paying selective attention to your bodily sensations, redirect your attention to the external environment. You are going to begin the simple and/or mundane task you've selected. After the five minutes end, jot down notes about your experience.

Table 8 Specific guidelines for focusing on mundane tasks

TASK SELECTED:	
Simple instructions: Once you set the timer for five minutes, begin your task. Note, your mind may drift and think about things or perhaps even start focusing on your bodily sensations again. Don't judge this. Simply redirect your focus back to the simple task or activity. Below are suggestions on how to use one or more of your five senses to help you stay focused on your task. Start by centering your attention on the minor details involved in the activity.	
Touch:	What does the task feel like in your hands? Notice the temperature of the item you are touching: is it cold, warm, hot? Notice how the surface of the item you are holding feels, thinking about the texture: is it smooth, rough, soft, hard? Notice the weight of the item in your hands: is it heavy or light? Be mindful of the tactile sensations in your hands as you engage in your activity.
Sight:	What do the items in your activity look like? What shapes are they? What colors do you see? What patterns do you see? What is the spatial arrangement of the different elements? What are the details you notice about each of the items you see? How does light play a role? Is the light natural or artificial? Do you notice any shadows or highlights? Is there movement or stillness in what you see?
Hearing:	What does the task sound like? Is it loud, soft, rhythmic or irregular? What are the primary sounds you hear? How would you describe these sounds? What are the secondary sounds you hear? Are there any variations in tone, pitch, volume or frequency? Does the sound remain steady or does it fluctuate over time?
Smell:	Do you notice any scents as you engage in this activity? What does it smell like? How would you describe these smells? Is it strong or mild and subtle? Does it vary in intensity? Does it shift or transform as you continue to experience it? Focus on the subtle nuances of the scent. Try to deconstruct the scent. What elements or ingredients stand out?
Taste:	What primary flavor do you notice? Are there multiple flavors? Try to notice the variations in flavor and different types of flavors. Is the taste strong or mild and subtle? Classify the taste into basic categories. Does the taste remain constant or does it evolve over time? Is the taste sweet, salty, sour or bitter? Is there an aftertaste and how long does it last?

Table 9 Thought record on 'Body focus' vs 'Mundane task focus'

Mundane task focus	**Observations during the focus period:** Were you able to stay focused on the task? How often did you notice any bodily sensations during this time? Was there any difference between the internal- and external-focused time periods?

You aren't done quite yet! I want you to practice this daily. You can also practice this with various bodily areas. Further, make this exercise more challenging as you grow in confidence by increasing the time in which you sustain focused attention.

Practicing these skills regularly can have two benefits. First, it helps you to recognize the power of your attention and focus. This will help you realize the more you focus on your bodily sensations, the more you notice any bodily changes and subsequently attribute these changes to you being in danger. Second, practicing this regularly can help you train yourself to be more intentional in (and ultimately have more influence over) how you direct your attention. Think of attention as a muscle. You want to strengthen it and this can be one step toward achieving that goal.

Exposure

Exposure is an evidence-based intervention used to treat all types of anxiety and anxiety-related disorders.[11,12,13] First, let's talk about what happens when we feel anxious or afraid of something. It is only natural to want to avoid the things in life that seem threatening. If a man with a knife started trailing you on the street, the appropriate, *adaptive* response would be to run in the other direction.

However, sometimes our mind inadvertently labels something as 'dangerous' when it is not. This is when the fear becomes maladaptive. Indeed, this mislabeling something as dangerous happens when one develops an irrational fear of *anything*, such as fear of dogs, fear of needles, fear of social situations, fear of heights or fear of flying. Many people with health anxiety specifically label bodily sensations and symptoms as dangerous due to the assumption that symptoms point to an immediate (heart attack) or eventual (cancer) catastrophe.

When we've determined something is dangerous, we either avoid it or engage in safety behaviors to cope with or manage the anxiety over the feared thing. For example, if we fear certain bodily sensations, we might refrain from working out or eating certain foods to avoid them, even if we have to give up things we love and/or know are good for us. Or, if we can't avoid the bodily sensations, we might engage in a safety behavior to keep us from perceived danger, such as checking our heart rate every five minutes so it doesn't get 'dangerously' high.

Interoceptive exposure

Exposure exercises can take many forms. Think of exposure as three main types:

1. imaginal exposures or repeatedly imagining feared scenarios
2. situational exposures or engaging in feared activities or scenarios in real life
3. interoceptive exposures or engaging in physical activities that intentionally bring on feared sensations
4. virtual reality exposure or exposing one to feared scenarios using virtual reality tools.

Interoceptive exposure helps you become more comfortable with and less afraid of bodily sensations, anxiety and uncertainty. It gives you a chance to learn that the catastrophic outcomes you fear with bodily sensations are unlikely and the discomfort associated with them is manageable and temporary. You are able to strengthen your sense of self-efficacy and coping skills when it comes to tolerating uncomfortable sensations. Importantly, lessening your fear of bodily sensations can also help you to rely less on safety behaviors and avoidance to cope with your fear. All of this helps break the vicious cycle of health anxiety.

More specifically, interoceptive exposure allows you to explore your fears by giving you the opportunity to assess their validity, through your own experience. Think of yourself like a scientist, testing your hypothesis or prediction about the catastrophic consequences of the feared bodily sensation, such as:

1 *My heart rate will get too high and I will have a heart attack.*
2 *Dizziness will lead me to faint and then I will hit my head and die.*
3 *Difficulty breathing will inevitably lead to suffocation and death.*
4 *Blurred vision is terrifying because it means I have a brain tumor.*

Further, interoceptive exposure can teach you distress tolerance skills, helping you see that you are more capable of tolerating anxiety than you assume. Again, although anxiety can certainly be uncomfortable and might *feel* dangerous, it is not actually harmful or dangerous. In this case, you are testing your prediction about the intolerability and danger of the anxiety itself, such as:

1 *I will not be able to manage the anxiety in the moment.*
2 *The anxiety symptoms will make me even more afraid and will ruin me.*
3 *The anxiety symptoms will never improve.*
4 *The anxiety symptoms will lead to catastrophic physical consequences.*
5 *The anxiety symptoms will cause me to go crazy or lose my mind.*

Ultimately, engaging in exposure exercises reshapes your beliefs and thoughts through your own experiences. I could preach to you all day long about how bodily sensations are tolerable, temporary and not automatically dangerous or indicative of a medical crisis or serious disease. But that isn't going to be nearly as impactful as it will be if you allow yourself to experience the feared sensations and come to your own conclusions about whether they are safe and tolerable.

Preparing for and planning exposure exercises

First, review all the steps involved in this process. Next, review the tips to optimize the benefits of exposure. Then we will plan your specific exposure tasks.

Importantly, in this section we have discussed exposure in terms of helping you face your feared bodily sensations. However, another component of exposure is *response prevention*, meaning that exposure tasks are tailored to prevent the use of your unhelpful safety behaviors. An inherent part of learning how to be less afraid of certain bodily sensations is to refrain from using safety behaviors during exposure exercises so that you can learn, through experience, that you don't need them.

In the next chapter, we will do an in-depth dive into using exposure and response prevention to help you reduce your use of safety and avoidant behaviors. In this section, however, we will be taking an initial 'baby step' toward becoming more comfortable with bodily sensations. You will then take the next step in Chapter 6 and continue exposure exercises while also refraining from using safety behaviors and avoidance. Let's get started with planning and implementing your exposure exercises. Below are a few key steps to follow.

Steps to selecting and implementing exposure tasks

Step 1: Obtain clearance from your healthcare provider. Typically speaking, these exercises are mild in intensity and do not pose any more risk than engaging in usual daily activities. However, some of these activities might be riskier if you have certain medical conditions (e.g. epilepsy and/or seizures, a heart condition, injuries, asthma, pregnancy). If you have a diagnosed medical condition and are unsure if these activities pose risk, consult with your doctor.

Step 2: Review Table 1 from earlier in this chapter (page 93) that lists many of the commonly experienced bodily sensations and symptoms. Make a list of any sensations that trigger anxiety for you. This will help inform the specific interoceptive exposure activities you will need to engage in to reduce your fear of the triggering bodily sensations.

Step 3: Take a look at Table 10 below that offers suggestions for interoceptive exercises based on the sensations that trigger your anxiety. Taking into consideration your feared sensations, make a note of the exercises that would be most beneficial. You may be able to simply look at this list and know exactly what to choose. However, if you are unsure of which ones bring anxiety, you could do a 'test run' with some of the exercises listed. Start by thinking about engaging in any of these exercises and if imagining yourself doing them makes you feel anxious at all, that might give you a good idea of what to include. You can also test this out further by trying some of these exercises and then making a note of the exercises that triggered anxiety.

Table 10 Examples of interoceptive exposure exercises

Feared bodily sensations or physiological experiences	Possible exposure activities
Feeling hot and stuffy, sweating, flushing, clamminess	Any intensive exercise such as running in place or running up and down stairs for at least two minutes, doing jumping jacks, going on a brisk walk or jog; drink a hot drink, sit in a hot, stuffy room, sauna or hot car, take a walk on a humid/hot day; sit while covered by a heavy coat or blanket.
Dizziness, light-headedness, faint feeling, blurred vision or feeling on the verge of loss of consciousness	Spin around in a swivel chair or spin in place for one minute; stare at bright light and then try to read something; shake head back and forth for 30 seconds and then look straight ahead; place head between legs for one minute; get up quickly from a sitting position; hold breath for 30 seconds.
Shortness of breath or difficulty breathing, tightening of the chest, smothering sensation	Hyperventilate (breathe in and out quickly at the rate of 100–120 breaths per minute) for one to five minutes or hyperventilate for one to five minutes while staring at a spiral or strobe light in a dark room; breathe through a straw while plugging your nose for two minutes; hold breath for 30 seconds to one minute; take one long, deep breath followed by several short breaths, breathing only from chest and maintaining a quick, shallow breathing pace.
Feeling unreal or in a dream-like state, feeling like one is losing control or going insane, depersonalization or derealization	Stare at yourself in mirror intently for three minutes, without shifting your gaze, or stare at a small dot on the wall or an optical illusion or rotating spiral for two minutes without shifting your gaze; hyperventilate (breathe in and out quickly at the rate of 100 to 120 breaths per minute) for one to five minutes or hyperventilate for one to five minutes while staring at a spiral or strobe light in a dark room; stare at a light on the ceiling for one minute and then read for one minute and repeat five to ten times.
Throat tightness or soreness, difficulty swallowing, choking sensation	Swallow quickly and repeatedly (ten times); clear throat multiple times in a row; wear a turtleneck; tighten a scarf or neck tie around neck for at least five minutes and then take a one-minute break (repeat three to five times).

Feared bodily sensations or physiological experiences	Possible exposure activities
Rapid or increased heart rate; chest pain, discomfort and/or tightness; heart palpitations	Any intensive exercise such as doing push-ups for one minute; running in place or up and down stairs for two minutes; doing aerobics; drink hot coffee; breathe through a straw while plugging nose for two minutes.
Tingling and numbness, trembling and shaking	Running in place or running up and down stairs; hyperventilate (breathe in and out quickly at the rate of 100 to 120 breaths per minute) for one to five minutes or hyperventilate for one to five minutes while staring at a spiral or strobe light in a dark room.
Nausea and vomiting	Spinning in place or spinning around in swivel chair for one minute; brush back of tongue with a toothbrush or hold tongue down with spoon for a few seconds or until trigger gag reflex (repeat 10 to 15 times); place head between legs for one minute.
Muscle tension, pain or tightness	While sitting down, tense or tighten all of your muscles for one minute; do a push-up and hold yourself up in this position for one minute and then rest and repeat five to ten times; lift weights with arms and/or legs for a lengthy period of time.

Step 4: Using the information you've jotted down thus far, write out a few exposure exercises you'd like to try out in the table below. Make a specific plan for when and how you will complete each exposure exercise.

Get started! Be sure to document all the details about the exposure task in the table below (the date, specific details about the activity and your anxiety level when it reaches its peak) as well as answer the reflection questions. This is a big part of the learning process.

Tips for selecting and implementing exposure exercises

Prior to getting started on your exposure exercises, read through this list of tips in order to maximize learning during this process.

- **Find the balance in terms of task difficulty:** Exposures should be both easy enough and hard enough. I'll explain. First, the overall goal of exposure is to face your fear to learn it is not as scary as you imagined and, ultimately, results in you being less afraid of that thing. Thus, for you to overcome your fears, you need to be sure the task brings at least *some* anxiety. Otherwise, what is the point? At the same time, you don't want the task to be too difficult or you may not follow through. Make sure that it is something you are likely to follow through with. It can help to start with a task that is anxiety-provoking but less intimidating and then work your way up to a more difficult one.

- **Exposures should be repeated often:** Practice your exercises often, ideally within a short timeframe. If you only do a task occasionally, it is harder to grow comfortable with the sensation. For example, if you engage in the task of running up and down your staircase, do it multiple times a day and continue throughout the week. Keep running until you notice your anxiety during this task consistently feels manageable. The more often you engage in these tasks, the more likely you will increase your distress tolerance and reduce your fear of these sensations.
- **Use your cognitive restructuring skills while engaging in exposure tasks:** Remember, it is helpful to challenge any unhelpful thoughts while you are completing exposure tasks. This will help to both reduce as well as cope with the anxiety you will experience during these tasks. As a starting place, you use the Socratic questions listed earlier in this chapter in Table 2 (page 97) to challenge any distorted thoughts related to the danger of bodily sensations.
- **Try to accept and tolerate the anxiety during the exposure tasks:** Learn how to cope with anxiety instead of trying to get rid of it. This is one of the goals of exposure in general, to increase your distress tolerance skills. We want you to learn, through personal experience, that anxiety, while annoying, is safe and tolerable. We also want you to increase your sense of confidence and self-efficacy as you learn to trust in your ability to tolerate anxiety.
- **Be aware of the inclination to use safety behaviors:** Be mindful of any temptation to engage in safety behaviors. As stated earlier, engaging in these brief exposure exercises is a first step in the process. We will prioritize *response prevention* more in the next chapter. For now, be mindful of any impulse or desire to engage in those familiar behaviors when you are feeling anxious during exposures (e.g. checking your heart rate). Whenever possible, refrain from the use of safety behaviors.

Danny's interoceptive exposure tasks

My client, Danny, believed an increased heart rate could trigger a heart attack, despite his doctor's reports of good cardiovascular health. He avoided caffeine, working out and any other activity that could increase his heart rate. He also engaged in safety behaviors. He checked his pulse multiple times a day, carried around a stethoscope and frequently went to urgent care when his heart rate seemed to get 'dangerously' high.

To help Danny reduce his fear of these bodily sensations, we started with a task that he thought would be manageable and not too intimidating. Danny walked up and down his staircase for two minutes and was only allowed to check his pulse twice (before, in this situation, he would have checked his pulse every 20 seconds or so). Afterward, he reflected on his experience. He then repeated this exposure task multiple times throughout the day for one week. As expected, his anxiety during this task decreased over time. More importantly, he learned that even though he did feel anxious, he was able to cope. In other words, it helped him to see that the anxiety itself wasn't his biggest enemy. His biggest enemies were his inaccurate assumptions that the symptoms were dangerous as well as his avoidance and safety behaviors.

Thought record of interoceptive exposure activities

Date/Time

October 22 at 8am

Exposure task

Run up and down stairs for two minutes

Highest level of anxiety (0–10)

8

Conclusions: Did anything bad happen? If not, was this different from what you expected? If so, how did you cope or deal with it? Were you able to tolerate your anxiety? What did you learn?

Nothing bad happened. There were times that I thought my heart might not be able to handle it as my heart rate increased but it turned out to be okay. When I was feeling stressed, I reminded myself that doctors have confirmed I don't have a heart condition so there isn't any evidence a rapid heart rate from anxiety/exercise could harm me.

Safety behaviors: Were you tempted to use any safety behaviors? If so, which ones? Were you able to refrain or reduce their use?

In the beginning, I had a hard time not checking my heart rate. The first time I did the exposure task, I still checked my heart rate about five times. However, each time I tried it and checked, it was less. I was able to reduce it every couple of days and eventually didn't check it at all.

How many times did you complete this task? Highest level of anxiety during the last task?

I did it three to four times per day for one week.

By the end, my anxiety was about a 2 or 3 at its peak

Now select your own interoceptive exposure exercises. Walk through each of the steps. Then begin your exercise. Remember, you'll want to repeat this process multiple times per day for a week or longer to improve your tolerance of, and ultimately reduce your fear of, these sensations. Do as many types of interoceptive exposure exercises as necessary. If you are triggered and anxious over multiple types of bodily sensations, engage in all of the exposure tasks that target each of your feared sensations.

References

1 McEwen BS. Central Role of the brain in stress and adaptation: Allostasis, biological embedding, and cumulative change. In: Fink G, ed. *Stress: Concepts, Cognition, Emotion, and Behavior*. Academic Press; 2016:39–55. <https://doi.org/10.1016/B978-0-12-800951-2.00005-4.>

2 Abramowitz JS, Braddock A. *Hypochondriasis and Health Anxiety*. Hogrefe Publishing GmbH; 2010. Accessed August 27, 2024. <https://pubengine2.s3.eu-central-1.amazonaws.com/previewwith99.110005/9781616763473_preview.pdf>

3 Billman GE. Homeostasis: The underappreciated and far too often ignored central organizing principle of physiology. *Frontiers in Physiology*. 2020;11(200). <https://doi.org/10.3389/fphys.2020.00200>

4 Billman GE. Homeostasis: The dynamic self-regulatory process that maintains health and buffers against disease. *Handbook of Systems and Complexity in Health.* Published online November 23, 2012:159–170. <https://doi.org/10.1007/978-1-4614-4998-0_10>
5 Sanderson C. *Health Psychology: Understanding the Mind–Body Connection,* 3rd Edition. Sage Publications; 2019. <https://www.proquest.com/docviewith2778441165?sourcetype=Other%20Sources>
6 Du X, Witthöft M, Zhang T, Shi C, Ren Z. Interpretation bias in health anxiety: A systematic review and meta-analysis – CORRIGENDUM. *Psychological Medicine.* Published online March 14, 2023:(1) 34–45. <https://doi.org/10.1017/s003329172300017x>
7 Marcus DK, Gurley JR, Marchi MM, Bauer C. Cognitive and perceptual variables in hypochondriasis and health anxiety: A systematic review. *Clinical Psychology Review.* 2007;27(2):127–139. <https://doi.org/10.1016/j.cpr.2006.09.003>
8 Shi C, Taylor S, Witthöft M, et al. Attentional bias toward health-threat in health anxiety: A systematic review and three-level meta-analysis. *Psychological Medicine.* 2022;52(4):604–613. <https://doi.org/10.1017/s0033291721005432>
9 Schwind J, Gropalis M, Witthöft M, Weck F. The effects of attention training on health anxiety: An experimental investigation. *Cognitive Therapy and Research.* 2015;40(2):245–255. <https://doi.org/10.1007/s10608-015-9745-x>
10 Wells A, Matthews G. *Attention and Emotion: A Clinical Perspective.* Psychology Press; 2016.
11 Ferrando C, Selai C. A systematic review and meta-analysis on the effectiveness of exposure and response prevention therapy in the treatment of Obsessive–Compulsive Disorder. *Journal of Obsessive-Compulsive and Related Disorders.* 2021;31:100684. <https://doi.org/10.1016/j.jocrd.2021.100684>
12 McLean CP, Levy HC, Miller ML, Tolin DF. Exposure therapy for PTSD: A meta-analysis. *Clinical Psychology Review.* 2022;91(91):102115. <https://doi.org/10.1016/j.cpr.2021.102115>
13 Garner LE, Steinberg EJ, McKay D. Exposure therapy. *Handbook of Cognitive Behavioral Therapy: Overview and Approaches (Vol 1).* Published online 2021:275–312. <https://doi.org/10.1037/0000218-010>

6

Stop using avoidance and safety behaviors

People with health anxiety tend to use both *avoidance* and *safety-seeking behaviors* as a coping mechanism when they are anxious about their health. Health-anxious people use these coping strategies in an attempt to reduce the anxiety they experience after being triggered by an internal (e.g. a new symptom or bodily sensation) or external event (e.g. a cancer story). All of these behaviors are used to reach one overarching goal: *to feel safer.* Ironically, however, although these behaviors might reduce anxiety in the moment, they ultimately increase anxiety over the long term. So, what do these behaviors look like? We will discuss avoidance and safety behaviors separately.

Please note that, as discussed in Chapter 1, health-anxious people who meet the criteria for Illness Anxiety Disorder typically fall into one of two categories: the *care-avoidant* or *care-seeking* subtype. Thus, as one might expect, care-avoidant subtypes are more likely to use avoidant behaviors and care-seeking subtypes are more likely to use safety behaviors such as reassurance-seeking from the healthcare system.

Avoidance

Avoidance, as you might expect, is when a person avoids anything that makes them feel anxious about their health. Avoidance can take many forms. Some people with health anxiety avoid getting physicals or regular check-ups at the doctor because they fear getting 'bad news' about their health. Or if they have a concerning symptom, they might avoid or put off getting it examined by a doctor, again because they fear being told that something is wrong. I had a client who was significantly overweight with a family history of heart disease. He had not gotten a physical or check-up in over ten years because he was terrified of what he might learn.

Others with health anxiety avoid reminders of certain diseases or sickness and death. They might avoid visiting people in the hospital, funerals or memorials, talking about death, reading obituaries, writing a will or reading books or watching movies or shows about illness and death. One of my clients avoided watching any movie or show related to cancer because her biggest fear was getting diagnosed with cancer. Some health-anxious people avoid anything they believe might lead them to contract an illness, such as airports, public restrooms, crowded places or visiting ill loved ones. I had a client who was terrified of using public restrooms because she feared she would somehow contract HIV or another sexually transmitted infection.

Lastly, many people with health anxiety avoid any activities that induce physiological sensations or changes in their physiological state because they mistakenly believe that the physiological sensations themselves are dangerous in some way. The most common example I have seen is avoiding exercise of any kind because of fears of an increased heart rate or altered breathing patterns. Some people might also avoid drinking caffeine, eating certain types of foods or having sex, as these can also lead to altered physiological states. The majority of my clients with health anxiety have stopped or changed their exercise habits because the physiological sensations brought them so much anxiety. One of my clients, a former marathon runner, had completely stopped going to the gym for over six months because it triggered so much health anxiety.

Why avoidance increases anxiety

Avoiding what makes us anxious about our health might reduce anxiety in the short term but it increases anxiety over the long term. Any time you avoid something, the fear of that thing grows more intense over time. This is true when it comes to any fear and health-related fears are no exception. For example, when we avoid exercise because we believe the physiological sensations pose some kind of a health threat, that 'threat' seems increasingly dangerous over time. The fear grows because we never give ourselves the chance to learn that the changes in our physiological state are not dangerous.

When we avoid the doctor because we are afraid of hearing 'bad news,' this fear increases and leads to more avoidance. But going to the doctor is an essential part of caring for our bodies. By avoiding the doctor, we never get the chance to learn that going to the doctor and learning we have a health issue does not put us in danger but actually makes us *safer* because then we can get the appropriate medical care.

Safety-seeking behaviors

Safety-seeking behaviors or safety behaviors are what health-anxious people *do* to reduce anxiety and uncertainty as well as to prevent their health fears from coming true. Think of safety behaviors as a subtle form of avoidance in which you put certain safeguards in place to prevent a potential medical crisis or medical disaster. For simplicity, we will break down safety behaviors into three main types: *reassurance-seeking, excessive checking* and *preventative.*

Let's start with *reassurance-seeking behaviors*. To deal with the stress of a new symptom or sensation, you collect information to assess what kind of danger you might be in. You might ask a friend or a family member what they think. '*Do you think this twitch is something neurological? Do I look flushed to you?*' Or you might go to primary care offices, urgent cares, hospitals or other medical facilities to consult with doctors and other medical professionals. You also might read all about the potential causes of the new symptom on the internet or in medical texts. And of course in today's world, all of this information is readily accessible. Your search history might include phrases like '*difficulty swallowing and esophageal cancer*' or '*less common symptoms of MS,*' or '*signs of unruptured aneurysm.*' Generally speaking, you seek reassurance from loved ones, physicians and the internet.

With *excessive checking behaviors*, you often monitor for symptoms, physical sensations or any kind of bodily function that might be 'concerning.' You might repeatedly poke or squeeze a part of your body or a new symptom. You might compare two sides of your body to identify any differences. You may inspect your feces or urine, check your heart rate, blood pressure, weight or lung capacity. Or perhaps you give yourself examinations of some kind, such as visual tests, neurological or cognitive tests or physical exertion tests. My clients have used a variety of clever and creative checking behaviors. One client would check for cancer signs by giving herself daily breast exams and another would search for blood in their stool with a toothpick. Those who feared a heart attack have checked their heart rate and blood pressure multiple times a day.

Preventative behaviors are attempts to prevent the possibility of future health problems. You might read incessantly about health recommendations or attend health classes or seminars. Or maybe you take a variety of supplements, work out religiously and/or go to great lengths to avoid a wide range of foods or drinks. To prevent consequences from any future health emergencies, you might ensure you have personal medical information, your phone, medical equipment or medication readily accessible at all times. Or you might prefer to have a safe person with you whenever possible or consistently keep loved ones updated on your whereabouts. When planning a long drive or trip to somewhere new, you might do research to ensure that the destination is located near an urgent care or hospital. Some of my clients have spent an exorbitant amount of time reading blogs, articles in medical journals and books. Other clients always made sure they brought a loved one with them when they went somewhere or were acutely aware of the nearest medical facility anytime they had to travel more than a few minutes away from home.

Why safety behaviors increase anxiety

Similar to avoidance, safety behaviors increase anxiety over time because we rely on them to achieve a sense of safety and rob ourselves of the opportunity to see that we never needed them to begin with. We might think, *Thank God I checked my pulse and stopped working out to slow down my heart rate. I would have had a heart attack.* But we never learn that we likely would not have had a heart attack, whether we checked our pulse a dozen times or none at all. The more we use safety behaviors, the more meaning and significance we give to them and, thus, the more dependent we become on them to feel safe. The cycle never ends and can become all-consuming.

Identifying your problematic behaviors

Similar to understanding problematic thoughts and beliefs, it is important that you understand problematic behaviors. Now that you know *what* avoidant and safety behaviors look like and *why* they make health anxiety worse, it is time to identify the behaviors you tend to use.

Table 1 Problematic coping behaviors

	Type	Examples
Avoidant behaviors	Avoid medical appointments	Avoid getting a physical or check-up; avoid going to doctor for new symptoms
	Avoid reminders of death and disease	Avoid hospitals or other medical facilities, funeral services, conversations about death, movies/shows about disease or death
	Avoid situations in which they may contract illness	Avoid using public restrooms or other shared spaces, crowded spaces like airports, visiting sick people, going to medical facilities in which sick people are encountered
	Avoid physiological sensations	Avoid exercise or any activity that brings on bodily sensations such as exercise or other activities that increase heart rate, consuming certain foods or drinks, hot temperatures, crowded spaces
	Type	**Examples**
Safety behaviors	Reassurance-seeking	Asking friends or family members about symptoms, repeatedly seeking reassurance from doctors and excessively searching for causes of symptoms on the internet.
	Excessive checking	Regularly checking the body for potential new symptoms or inspecting old symptoms (e.g. checking moles or lumps, assessing heart rate, lung capacity), and giving oneself various tests or examinations.
	Preventative	Read incessantly about health recommendations, obsessively monitor food and drink consumption, ensure that medical facilities, medical equipment or people are nearby in case of a medical crisis.

when you are anxious about your health. Review the summary table below and make note of any avoidant behaviors and/or safety behaviors that resonate with you. Awareness is the first step.

Let's take note of your common behaviors. First, after reviewing the list above, make a list of all the things you do (or don't do) when you are anxious about your health. Next, review your behaviors over the past couple of weeks. This will help you get into the habit of noticing how this process plays out. For the past two weeks, note down any situations, your anxious thoughts and subsequent behaviors. This will help you develop awareness of your behavioral patterns.

Table 2 My problematic safety behaviors and/or avoidant behaviors

My safety behaviors	My avoidant behaviors

Table 3 Record of situations, anxious thoughts and behavioral responses

Date & situation or trigger & level of anxiety (1–10)	Anxious thoughts/ thinking errors	What I did/didn't do (i.e. safety behaviors and avoidance)
11/15 Noticed a skin blemish on my arm Anxiety (8/10)	What if it is melanoma? Level of concern (9/10)	Began picking at my skin and picked at it 10–15 times throughout the rest of the day (i.e. excessive checking) Started googling symptoms of melanoma (i.e. reassurance-seeking) Asked my girlfriend several times throughout the day if she thinks it's cancer (i.e. reassurance-seeking)

Taking a more balanced approach

Health consciousness is not bad. It is prudent and necessary to see a doctor if you have a new lump or a changing mole. Women should give themselves breast exams once a month. And it is good to work out and make informed, healthy decisions about the things you eat and drink. These are all necessary ways of taking care of yourself. However, when the things you do to manage your health become excessive and of constant dire significance, you have slipped into the realm of safety behaviors. It is one thing to take reasonable steps to optimize your health and live a balanced lifestyle. It is entirely another if you believe the daily use of all of these behaviors is what stands between life and death.

Imagine your health-related behaviors as being on a spectrum (see diagram below). On one side, you have complete avoidance. On the other side of the spectrum is the excessive use of safety behaviors that we've been talking about.

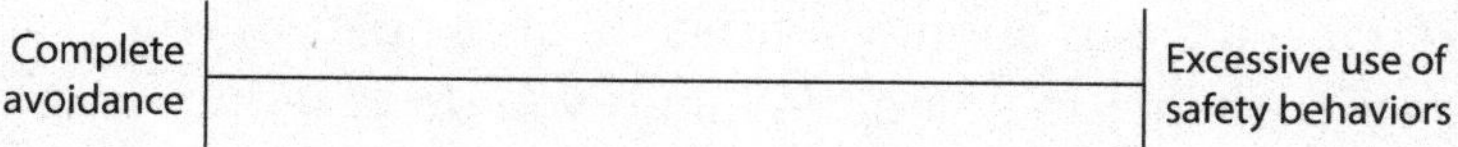

Think of safety behaviors and avoidance as being the two extremes in terms of how one manages their health. In other words, one extreme is micromanaging your health and the other extreme is not managing or minimally managing your health. Both of these extremes are, of course, just different ways of coping with health anxiety and neither one of them is good for you. The goal is to take a more balanced approach when it comes to your health.

A balanced approach sits in the middle of this spectrum, between these two extremes. So, for example, you go to the doctor for persistent symptoms, get all the recommended check-ups and screenings or tests, take the necessary or recommended vitamins and supplements, exercise regularly, eat a balanced and nutritious diet, prioritize your sleep and refrain from smoking or excessive alcohol intake. Further, if you have a medical condition, you make sure you are following all of your doctor's orders and recommendations to effectively manage the disease.

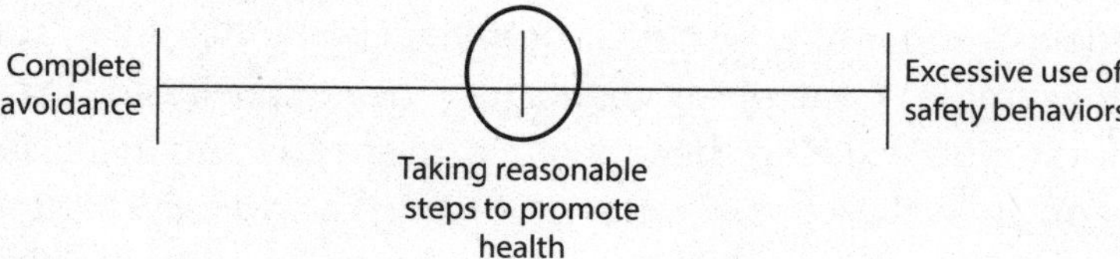

However, to stay in the middle of the spectrum, you'll have to learn how to live with a little bit of uncertainty when it comes to your health. In this chapter, I will teach you several cognitive and behavioral techniques to help you learn to live near the middle of this spectrum when it comes to your health-related behaviors.

The cost–benefit analysis

Exploring the impact of avoidance and safety behaviors

You might be aware of some of the ways your avoidance and/or safety behaviors are negatively impacting your life. Perhaps you recognize that after spending an hour or two googling symptoms, you only feel more anxious and stressed. However, there is a reason you do these things when you feel anxious about your health. Some part of you believes there are advantages to doing the things you do to reduce your health anxiety or, quite frankly, you wouldn't do them.

It can be helpful to explore both the costs and benefits of a given behavior to see just how much your behaviors are helping and/or hurting you. This can serve several useful purposes. First, it can help you identify your motivations or reasons for using certain behaviors, which gives us the opportunity to evaluate the validity of these reasons. The cost–benefit analysis also helps you to better understand the consequences, or costs, of using avoidance and/or safety behaviors. Lastly, this exercise gives you the opportunity to think of a more adaptive behavior that you can use to replace your unhelpful behavior. We are then able to evaluate the perceived costs and benefits of using the new, adaptive behavior.

Sometimes, when I introduce this exercise, my health-anxious clients will say they don't think it is necessary because they already know their behavior is problematic. However, after doing the exercise and digging a little deeper, we uncover some motivational influences they didn't even know about. In other words, they didn't realize they had made assumptions about their behaviors being helpful in some way. For example, some of my clients have been convinced that their body monitoring will help them detect cancer early and increase their chances of survival. However, after evaluating the impact of these behaviors, they see more clearly that their behavior is hurting them much more than it is helping them. They also are able to get a glimpse of how life could be if they started using more adaptive behaviors.

Daniel's safety behavior of frequent medical visits

A common coping strategy I have seen my clients use when they worry about their health is to frequently seek reassurance from doctors. Let's use an example of one of my former clients, Daniel. The whole situation went a little something like this:

1. Daniel noticed heart palpitations.
2. Daniel felt anxious because he thought something was wrong.
3. Daniel went to the doctor.
4. The doctor examined him, ran a test or two and said he was fine.
5. Daniel felt less anxious and went home.
6. Daniel noticed heart palpitations again two days later.
7. Daniel was even more anxious (this time something must be *really* wrong).
8. Daniel headed to the urgent care.
9. Urgent care sent him home with the same conclusion.
10. Daniel felt a little better but had more anxiety than before, as he began to conclude the doctors were mistaken.

This cycle continued over the next few weeks Daniel showed back up at urgent care and his doctor's office a few more times. All exams and test results revealed no concerns.

Daniel's cost–benefit analysis

Daniel genuinely believed that going to the doctor or urgent care every week was helping him in some way. The cost–benefit analysis helped him to take a step back to look at the big picture of how this behavior was impacting his life. Below are the results of Daniel's cost–benefit analysis.

Steps to conduct a cost–benefit analysis

1. Label the maladaptive safety behavior or coping strategy, in this case *frequently going to the doctor.*
2. List all of the advantages/benefits of the maladaptive coping strategy.
3. List all of the disadvantages/costs of the maladaptive coping strategy. This section can help you see just how much this behavior is negatively impacting your life.
4. Go back up to the advantages of the maladaptive coping strategy and give them a thorough, critical analysis. Look for any thinking errors or biases in the logic of these reasons and then write out your reframe. This is an essential step because you likely are assuming

some of these are advantages when they aren't necessarily. Ask yourself, is this really an advantage?

Daniel's maladaptive coping strategy: *Frequently going to the doctor.*

Advantages of maladaptive coping strategy:

- Can be assured that everything is okay when the doctor says the symptom is not indicative of a serious issue. *REFRAME: Sometimes I feel reassured... but even then the reassured feeling only lasts a little while. Also, there are a lot of times that I do NOT feel reassured and am unsatisfied because I don't get the answers I am seeking.*
- While there, I can ask questions about other health concerns to gather information and follow recommendations regarding other potential health issues. *REFRAME: This doesn't usually work out anyway. The doctor doesn't have time to answer all of my questions and I usually end up not getting the answers I want about everything and, therefore, feel more confused and anxious than before.*
- It is a form of preventative care in that it might help me identify a disease in the early stages. Thus, it could prevent the disease from spreading and killing me. *REFRAME: It is possible that going to the doctor every week could help me find something early. But this has never happened to me. It is usually nothing or a mild sickness. Plus, I could still identify a disease in the early stages without having to be paranoid or go in every week. I could take reasonable steps to take care of my health and catch something early.*
- If I suddenly have a medical emergency at that moment, at least I am around medical professionals to keep me from dying. *REFRAME: But what are the chances that something life threatening happens while I am at the doctor? This has never happened.*

Disadvantages of maladaptive coping strategy:

- *I spend several hours a week dealing with medical visits, making calls for appointments and dealing with bills and questions. It takes time away from other things that are important and give me pleasure (hobbies, working out, work, friends, family).*

- *Embarrassed by my behavior, I often hide what I am doing from my family, friends.*
- *I have paid over a thousand dollars in copayments and deductibles for procedures that were likely not even necessary.*
- *It is a pain and inconvenience.*
- *I am often not reassured and even feel more anxious afterward sometimes. The process can feel very debilitating, depressing and hopeless.*
- *I feel out of control—seeking answers that I never get.*
- *It has put a strain on my social relationships—spouse and friends get tired of going through the emotional roller coaster with me.*

Steps to conduct a cost–benefit analysis (continued)

1 Come up with a more adaptive coping strategy (*taking reasonable steps to promote health and accepting uncertainty*). In this case, we have Daniel take reasonable steps to manage his health (i.e. healthy eating, sleep and exercise as well as following general medical recommendations and guidelines). However, beyond taking those reasonable steps, we want Daniel to learn how to accept and live with some uncertainty about bodily sensations and his health.
2 List out all of the advantages/benefits of using the more adaptive behavior. This can help you see how life could look different.
3 List out all of the disadvantages/costs of using the adaptive coping strategy. This will help you identify any potential barriers or challenges to making this change so that you can plan, prepare and problem-solve for those barriers.

Daniel's new, adaptive coping strategy: *Taking reasonable steps to manage my health and accepting some uncertainty.*

Advantages of adaptive coping strategy:

- *I will be able to use the extra time and energy (i.e. five+ hours each week going to the doctor) to play golf, work out and do other activities that bring me fulfillment.*

- *I won't have to manage difficult emotions on a regular basis (embarrassment in front of family, anger at doctors, anxiety over not getting the answers I want).*
- *My relationship with my wife would improve. She gets frustrated with me because she has to make up for the time I spend going to doctor appointments, as she has to pick up the slack with the kids, responsibilities around the house. Also, she wouldn't be so frustrated about me spending so much money on medical visits.*
- *I would have extra money without all the medical expenses. I can spend my extra money on something fun like going out for family weekend getaways and dinner with my wife and happy hour with my friends and coworkers. Also, I wouldn't feel so bad about using the money.*
- *My kids would feel safer because they wouldn't hear me talking about my health concerns/doctor visits with my wife all of the time and see me often coming home from the doctor or urgent care.*
- *Acceptance can bring freedom from the anxiety involved in seeking out certainty when it is not possible to be certain that I will never get a serious disease.*

Disadvantages of adaptive coping strategy:

- It seems like an impossible task. I have been doing this for so long and can't imagine being able to stop. *REFRAME: Anytime someone tries to do something new or different, it is a challenge. That does not make it impossible. I have been able to make other positive changes in my life, like going back to school to start a whole new career later in life or moderate my drinking. I can use these same transferable skills to help me commit to this too. I will take baby steps and get support/encouragement from my therapist, wife and best friend to help me see it through.*
- It will be hard work and require concerted effort to refrain from running to the doctor for every minor ache or pain. I will also have to endure an increase in anxiety when I begin to work on it because it will feel wrong/unnatural to give into the urge to go to the doctor. *REFRAME: Again, any real change takes hard work and commitment. I can seek help from loved ones and my therapist to hold me accountable to follow through. I also will have to remind myself that it is good to get more comfortable with anxiety*

because I need to learn that I can tolerate anxiety and uncertainty. My therapist is always telling me that the better I get at that, the less I will see it as the 'big, scary monster in the closet.' Tolerating anxiety is part of the process of getting better.

- There is a possibility that by not going to the doctor a lot, I could miss something serious and get really sick and die. *REFRAME: This is likely distorted thinking. It is not that simple. If there is a symptom that is concerning and doesn't go away or worsens, of course I will go to the doctor. I'm just not going to the doctor for every single bodily sensation.*

Steps to conduct a cost–benefit analysis (continued)

4 After you are done with all of these steps, take a minute to look over all of the evidence, including the reframes. Spend a little time to sit with all of the information. Essentially, you are taking a 'helicopter view' or 'bird's eye view' of everything.

5 After your thorough review, start with the maladaptive strategy (*frequently going to the doctor*) and ask yourself: if you had 100 points to divide up between advantages and disadvantages of the maladaptive coping strategy, how many points would you give the advantages section and how many points would you give the disadvantages section?

6 Now, go to the adaptive coping strategy (*taking reasonable steps to promote health and accepting uncertainty*) and ask yourself the same question. How many points would you give the disadvantages section and how many points would you give the advantages section?

Daniel's results

After completing the cost–benefit analysis, Daniel was able to see just how much his coping strategy of frequently going to the doctor was negatively impacting his life. He also was able to get a glimpse of how life could be better if he chose to replace this behavior with a more adaptive one. As you can see, after Daniel's thorough analysis and review of all of the costs and benefits of his maladaptive behavior (*frequently going to the doctor*), he determined that the costs or disadvantages (70) heavily outweighed the benefits or advantages (30). Further, in reviewing all of the costs and benefits of using a more adaptive behavior (*taking reasonable steps to promote his health and accepting uncertainty*), he determined that the benefits (65) outweighed the costs (35).

Overall, this activity helped Daniel to see his behavior more clearly than he did before. He was able to take a 'helicopter view' or 'bird's eye view' of how what he does when he is anxious about his health impacts his life. You can use this strategy to examine a variety of maladaptive coping strategies or even to examine the utility of holding maladaptive beliefs. Below are a few examples of other maladaptive coping behaviors you might evaluate in a cost–benefit analysis.

Examples of maladaptive coping strategies

- Searching online about symptoms and bodily sensations
- Reassurance-seeking from loved ones
- Excessive use of preventive behaviors
- Avoiding doctors, medical tests/exams or reminders of disease or death (movies, books, conversations, news articles)
- Engaging in excessive worry about health-related issues

Let's give it a try! Following my tips and Daniel's example, complete a cost–benefit analysis of your own problematic behavior. Start by examining the costs and benefits of the behavior(s) that are most problematic in your life. Further, Daniel's analysis is of one very specific type of reassurance-seeking, excessive medical appointments. However, you can be more general if you'd prefer. For example, you could do a cost–benefit analysis of all types of reassurance-seeking behaviors.

Exposure and response prevention

In Chapter 5, you learned the evidence for and rationale behind exposure therapy and how to plan and implement interoceptive exposure exercises to reduce your fear of bodily sensations as well as build confidence in your ability to tolerate anxiety and uncertainty over feared bodily sensations. This chapter will help you continue to practice facing feared bodily sensations (as well as learn how to face feared situations) but you will also learn how to refrain from using safety behaviors through a systematic, step-by-step process. Thus, in this chapter you will be engaging in both *exposure* and *response prevention.*

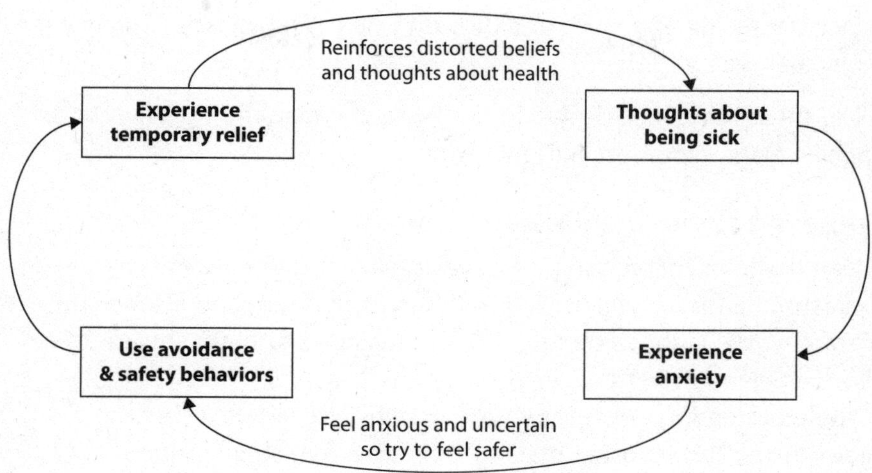

Remember, safety behaviors and avoidance only further reinforce dysfunctional beliefs about health (as illustrated in the diagram). You use these maladaptive coping mechanisms, but they become a vicious cycle by reinforcing the idea that these behaviors are necessary for your sanity and survival. By refraining from these behaviors, you learn that: (1) you can tolerate the anxiety and uncertainty associated with bodily sensations/ health concerns; and (2) you are unlikely to experience a catastrophic health outcome because you don't use a particular safety behavior.

To accomplish this, we will use what is called an exposure hierarchy or fear hierarchy. An exposure hierarchy is a series of exposure tasks placed in hierarchical order, typically including around 10–20 tasks. The key is to face feared sensations and situations without using safety behaviors. We begin with the least-distressing tasks at the bottom of the hierarchy (ideally a task that prompts around 40/100 subjective units of distress) and work our way up to the most difficult or distressing (a task that prompts 100/100 subjective units of distress). This allows you to build confidence as you work your way through to the top.

Types of exposure tasks

1. imaginal exposures or repeatedly imagining feared scenarios
2. situational exposures or engaging in feared activities or scenarios in real life
3. interoceptive exposures or engaging in physical activities that intentionally bring on feared sensations.

4 virtual reality exposure or exposing one to feared scenarios using virtual reality tools

All of these may be included in the hierarchy, depending on your specific fears, behaviors and intentions.

Preparing for your exposure hierarchy

Given the idiosyncratic nature of your fears and behaviors, your exposure hierarchy will look very different than anyone else's exposure hierarchy. We want to be focused and targeted to make this exercise more efficient and effective.

Before creating items for your hierarchy, we will first need to brainstorm. This involves making three lists, which will ultimately aid you in developing exposure items that target your specific thoughts and behaviors. I will walk you through this entire process with an example from one of my former clients, Ashonte.

Please note, for those of you who engage in healthcare avoidance, you will see an example of an exposure hierarchy that targets healthcare avoidance in Chapter 8.

List 1: Feared consequences

This will perhaps be a shorter list and fairly straightforward. We all have underlying core fears that fuel our health anxiety. Think about what it is that you ultimately fear. I've included a table of examples below. My biggest fear was always dying young from a serious disease. Sure, I didn't like the idea of being debilitated and dependent on others but that didn't terrify me nearly as much as the possibility of getting diagnosed with a terminal illness and being told I have months to live. More specifically, I feared a terminal cancer diagnosis and/or a progressive degenerative

Table 4 Examples of feared consequences

• Being diagnosed with a serious illness and living with guilt and regret because of beliefs that it could have been prevented somehow
• Becoming debilitated or incapacitated due to a sudden medical crisis, serious disease or severe mental illness
• Becoming isolated or dependent on others and unable to care for oneself
• Experiencing physical and emotional pain from having a medical crisis, disease or severe mental illness
• Dying from a sudden medical crisis or serious disease
• 'Going crazy' or losing connection to reality due to severe mental illness

disease like early-onset dementia or Alzheimer's. In thinking about your core fears, try to be specific, as the goal is to facilitate identifying the most relevant exposure exercises possible.

Ashonte's feared consequences

Ashonte ultimately feared dying and leaving her loved ones behind. She specifically feared some sort of medical crisis that would either result in sudden death or lead to the discovery of a serious illness. For example, she worried that she would faint, leading to one of two outcomes: (1) she would hit her head from fainting, which would lead to a serious brain injury and kill her; or (2) she would be sent to the hospital and would discover that she had a brain tumor or some other deadly disease. Ashonte also worried about getting diagnosed with and ultimately dying from a terrible disease like cancer.

List 2: Feared situations and cues

Bearing in mind your feared consequences, what types of specific situations trigger you? Are there certain physiological sensations that make you think the feared consequence is about to happen? Are there thoughts that pop into your head that make you anxious? What environments make you particularly anxious and remind you of your core fears? For example, do certain situations, circumstances or reminders of disease and death trigger your health anxiety? Reviewing your worksheet in Chapter 2 on internal and external triggers might help you identify feared situations or cues. I've provided a brief list of examples in Table 5.

Table 5 Examples of feared situations and cues

Internal fear cues/triggers: (physical sensations; thoughts)	**External fear cues/triggers:** (circumstances; places; reminders of death and disease)
Recurring and/or intrusive thoughts about death, disease, suffering physiological sensations, such as dizziness, sweatiness, trembling, blurred vision, breathlessness or labored breathing, feeling hot or sweaty, feeling trapped or cramped	Certain stores, driving, crowded places, hospital or other medical facilities or specific departments (oncology department), funeral homes, cemeteries, watching certain movies or shows, books, articles or social media accounts, public spaces with potential germs, certain sounds (coughing) or sights (a sick person)

Ashonte's feared situations and cues

Given that one of Ashonte's biggest fears was fainting, she feared going to stores or running other errands by herself. For example, she worried about going grocery shopping alone because she was afraid that if she fainted, there would be no one to keep her from collapsing to the floor and hitting her head. She also worried that she wouldn't be able to get medical help in time if she was shopping alone.

Ashonte's biggest feared internal cues or triggers related to fainting and included any sensations she thought suggested she was about to faint, such as blurred or spotty vision, dizziness or feeling weak or lightheaded. Her biggest feared external cues or triggers included being alone while shopping or driving.

Ashonte also feared getting diagnosed with cancer. External cues or triggers related to this fear included learning about other people's cancer stories or going to the doctor or any situation in which she could potentially receive terrible news about her health, even when she was simply getting a routine physical or mammogram. She also became anxious anytime she was triggered by internal cues, such as when she had intrusive thoughts and images of her dying from cancer or when she noticed new symptoms she believed were signs of cancer, such as a changing mole, a new lump or bump or body aches or pains.

List 3: Safety behaviors and avoidance

We have covered your core fears and the specific internal and external cues that trigger these fears. Now I want you to think about what you *do* (or *don't do*) when these fears are triggered. In other words, when you become anxious about your health, what actions or inactions do you take to either cope with the anxiety or prevent a feared medical catastrophe? This list isn't new to you since we covered this at the beginning of the chapter. However, I want you to be targeted in considering the behaviors (or avoidance) you engage in as it relates to the underlying core fears and triggers you just identified. For a more detailed list, revisit Table 1.

Ashonte's safety behaviors and avoidance

Coping with fainting cues. To cope with her fear of fainting in the store or fainting while driving, Ashonte often brought a 'safe person' with her when she went out, typically her sister or her boyfriend. If a safe person wasn't available when she needed to go to the store, she would often avoid it altogether or would find another way to get what she needed (e.g. having groceries delivered).

At times, she pushed through and forced herself to go even without a safe person. However, during these solo errands, she would regularly assess her 'fainting vulnerability' by checking in with her body to search for signs of dizziness or weakness. She would also try to walk closer to one side of the aisle so she could immediately reach out and grab onto one of the shelves if she started to feel faint. When Ashonte had to drive alone, she would drive slowly by the edge of the highway so she would be able to immediately pull over if she thought she might faint. She also paid very close attention to her vision and sense of strength while driving, to promote early detection of a fainting spell so she could pull over.

Coping with cancer cues. First, if she was anticipating a visit to the doctor or awaiting test results, she would read extensively about the odds of getting certain types of cancer or the risk factors for cancer. She would also ask her boyfriend and friends about whether they thought she was at high risk for getting diagnosed with cancer. She also consumed a lot of content on social media about cancer from doctors and people living with cancer to gather information about common symptoms to watch for or how to prevent certain types of cancer.

Table 6 Ashonte's summary of feared consequences, fear cues and coping behaviors

Feared consequences
• Dying from a sudden medical crisis, such as fainting and hitting head • Dying from an underlying disease, such as cancer • Ultimately, she feared dying because she feared leaving loved ones behind
Feared situations & cues or triggers

• Going shopping alone due to fear of fainting
• Driving due to fear of fainting
• Going to the doctor for any reason
• Awaiting the results of a test
• Hearing someone else's scary cancer story
• Reading online about rates of different types of cancer
• Intrusive images or thoughts about having cancer
• Symptoms presumed to be related to:
  ○ Fainting (blurred/spotty vision, dizziness, fatigue or light headedness)
  ○ Cancer (changing moles, new lumps or bumps, body aches or pains)

Table 6 (*Continued*)

Safety behaviors & avoidance
• Bring a 'safe person' with her to the store to prevent injury from fainting • Avoid going to store and ordering groceries online instead • When at store, hyper focus on body to look for any signs of fainting • Walk close to the aisle while at store to grab onto something if feeling faint • Drive slowly and in slow lane so that can pull over if going to faint • While driving, hyper focus on body to look for any signs of fainting • Avoid routine medical appointments because of fear of being told she has cancer • Avoid reading or watching anything related to cancer (e.g. news articles, movies)

It's your turn! Similar to Ashonte's example, make a table that includes a list for each of these three categories. You will then draw from your table and use it as inspiration for creating an exposure hierarchy.

Table 7 My summary of feared consequences, fear cues and coping behaviors

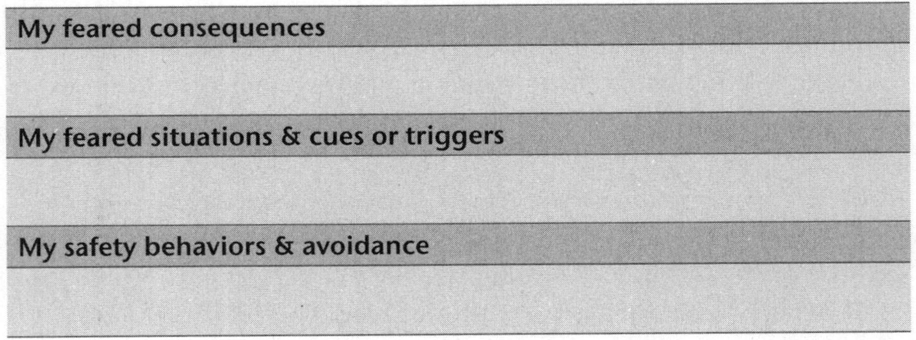

My feared consequences
My feared situations & cues or triggers
My safety behaviors & avoidance

Once you have brainstormed and developed your lists, create the hierarchy. Again, we will include around 10–20 items that we will place in order, starting with the easiest task (40/100 SUDS) and working our way up to the hardest task (100/100 SUDS). Think of the process as taking baby steps that will get more challenging as you progress through the steps and increase your confidence. Exposure items could be situational, imaginal or interoceptive. The goal is to face situations, sensations or images that provoke your health anxiety, while refraining from the use of safety behaviors. See Ashonte's exposure hierarchy (Table 11) for a detailed illustration.

Table 8 Ashonte's exposure hierarchy

Task #	Ashonte's exposure hierarchy	SUDS
12	Will drive 45 minutes to my sister's house (no safety behaviors allowed). I am not allowed to focus on my body, drive slowly or pull over. I must drive at the speed limit and in the middle lane. (*I will focus on the external environment instead of my body by listening to my audiobook*).	100/100
11	Schedule and attend my annual mammogram (no safety behaviors allowed). While waiting for results, I will refrain from seeking reassurance from loved ones, looking up information on cancer, and watching or reading about people's cancer stories on social media.	95/100
10	Shop at a store for 30 minutes (no safety behaviors allowed). I am not allowed to bring a safe person or my phone into the store with me. I am not allowed to search my body for symptoms and must walk in the middle of the aisle (*I will use cognitive restructuring/attention control exercises to focus on the external environment instead of my body*).	90/100
9	Schedule and attend my biannual physical (no safety behaviors allowed). While waiting for results, I will refrain from seeking reassurance from loved ones, looking up information on cancer, and watching or reading about people's cancer stories on social media.	85/100
8	Will drive 15 minutes to the nearest grocery store (no safety behaviors allowed). I am not allowed to focus on my body, drive slowly or pull over. I must drive at the speed limit and in the middle lane. (*I will focus on the external environment instead of my body, by listening to my audiobook*).	80/100
7	Watch a movie about someone with cancer all the way through. I am not allowed to distract myself or tune out while watching if it becomes overwhelming. (*I will use cognitive restructuring exercises to challenge any unhelpful thoughts that come up during this exercise.*)	75/100
6	Shop at a store for 15 minutes to buy one item (no safety behaviors allowed). I am not allowed to bring a safe person or phone into the store with me. I cannot search my body for symptoms and must walk in the middle of the aisle (*I will use cognitive restructuring/attention control exercises to focus on the external environment instead of my body*).	70/100

Table 8 (*Continued*)

Task #	Ashonte's exposure hierarchy	SUDS
5	Will drive five minutes to nearest gas station and back (no safety behaviors allowed). I am not allowed to focus on my body, drive slowly or pull over. I must drive at the speed limit and in the middle lane. (*I will focus on the external environment, instead of my body, by listening to my favorite playlist of songs.*)	65/100
4	Will do an imaginal exercise about getting a cancer diagnosis. I will write out a scenario about walking into the doctor's office to get the results of a scan and receiving a cancer diagnosis. I will imagine taking in the diagnosis information, telling my loved ones and beginning treatment.	55/100
3	Will shop at a store for five minutes to buy one item (no safety behaviors allowed). I am not allowed to bring a safe person or my phone into the store with me. I am not allowed to search my body for symptoms. I am not allowed to walk close to the side of the aisle so I can grab onto something if I faint. (*I will use cognitive restructuring/attention control exercises to focus on the external environment instead of bodily sensations.*)	50/100
2	Read a brief article about cancer in one sitting (one page or several paragraphs). I am not allowed to distract myself or tune out while reading if it becomes overwhelming. (*I will use cognitive restructuring exercises to challenge any unhelpful thoughts that come up during this exercise.*)	45/100
1	Engage in imaginal exposure exercise: will write out a scenario about going to a store alone for 30 minutes without using any safety behaviors (i.e. no phone, walk in middle of aisle). I will imagine experiencing fainting symptoms and continuing to shop until the symptoms fade.	35/100

Note that when Ashonte completed the task of shopping at the store, she got a ride with her boyfriend but her boyfriend did not go into the store with her. For those items, we were specifically working on the safety behavior of shopping by herself (and not driving by herself). In other words, in this hierarchy, we worked on her fear of fainting while driving and her fear of fainting while shopping separately.

Further, in this exposure example we included items related to both Ashonte's core fears: cancer and fainting. However, for simplicity purposes, you can choose to focus on one at a time. For example, you may want to create an exposure hierarchy of ten items to specifically target your fear of fainting first. You could then do a separate hierarchy for cancer.

Now, it is your turn! Below is a list of the steps for creating your own exposure hierarchy. I've also included some tips for successful development and implementation of the exposure hierarchy.

Steps to designing and implementing an exposure hierarchy

Step 1: As in Chapter 5, if you plan to include any interoceptive exposure items in your hierarchy, you will want to obtain clearance from your healthcare provider. Although interoceptive exercises are mild in intensity, they might be risky for those with certain medical conditions. If you have a diagnosed medical condition and/or are unsure if these activities pose a risk to you, consult with your doctor.

Step 2: Carefully review the list of tips for optimizing the development and implementation of exposure tasks before you get started (see list in Table 9 below). Do this *before* developing or completing the tasks. It will help you develop items that most effectively target your problematic thoughts and behaviors. It will also teach you key strategies to help you get through the exposure tasks, particularly when it gets difficult.

Step 3: Review your table that lists your (1) *feared consequences;* (2) *feared situations and cues or triggers*; as well as (3) the *safety behaviors and avoidance behaviors* you engage in. Using your table as inspiration and Ashonte's exposure hierarchy as an example, make a list of 10 to 20 different exposure tasks (with varying levels of difficulty) you will engage in that specifically target your feared situations and safety behaviors. You can accomplish this step in a couple of different ways.

Option 1: Identify and list items one by one in order of difficulty. You can start from the bottom and identify an item that is around 40/100 SUDS. You then continue to develop each new item as you work your way up the hierarchy, typically moving up in SUDS by about five or ten points with each task (e.g. find an exposure item that is 40/100, then 45/100 and so on).

Option 2: Make a large list of different exposure tasks you can engage in without ranking them. You then, subsequently, assign a SUDS to each one and put them in their respective places on the hierarchy. Again, items with a lower SUDS rating (lowest at around 40/100) will be placed at the bottom of the hierarchy and items with higher SUDS ratings will be placed at the top of the hierarchy, the most difficult being 100/100.

Notably, when developing items, consider your use of safety behaviors. Exposure has been used in different ways and there is considerable debate in the field about whether (and how) to permit the use of safety behaviors during exposure tasks.[1] Ideally, you completely refrain from the use of safety behaviors during exposure tasks, as this maximizes learning. However, it may be too overwhelming to do an exposure task without any coping aids. If this is the case, you can choose to start by allowing yourself to use safety behaviors on a minimal basis, with the goal of eventually refraining from all safety behavior use as you work your way to the top of the hierarchy. Again, keep in mind that your exposure hierarchy will be different from anyone else's, given your unique fears and behaviors. An item that is a 45/100 SUDS for you might be a 75/100 for someone else.

Step 4: Now that you have completed your hierarchy, it's time to plan the specifics! Commit to when and how you will complete each exposure exercise. My clients and I typically only make a specific plan for the tasks they will complete that week. It is helpful to include information on your predictions, potential challenges and strategies

Table 9 Weekly exposure planning log (with Ashonte's example)

Exposure tasks to complete this week (& date)	What do I predict will happen?	Anticipated challenges or potential barriers to task completion	How I will address challenges to ensure task completion
Will drive five minutes to gas station alone (#5) Date to be completed: 10/23	Prediction #1: I might faint while driving and could crash. Prediction #2: I won't be able to refrain from using all of my safety behaviors.	It might be too hard for me to not use my safety behaviors, especially the safety behavior of checking my body for signs of fainting. I may get too scared and quit in the middle of it.	To help me refrain from hyper focusing on my body, I will redirect my focus to the external environment (e.g. will listen to my audiobook). Will also use critical thinking to challenge thoughts: remind myself that there is no basis for my fears—I have never fainted before so I am highly unlikely to start fainting during this one particular drive.

Exposure tasks to complete this week (& date)	What do I predict will happen?	Anticipated challenges or potential barriers to task completion	How I will address challenges to ensure task completion
Shop at a store alone for 15 minutes (#6) Date to be completed:10/25	Prediction #1: Will start to faint and won't be able to grab the shelves because I can't use the safety behavior of walking near the side of the aisle. Prediction #2: I won't be able to handle the anxiety that comes with not being able to use any safety behaviors.	It will be hard to shop without using my safety behaviors (e.g. middle of aisle, focusing on body, safe person with me). It will be scary and I will be thinking of my worst fears—that I will faint, go to the hospital and find out terrible news.	To help me push through my fears and complete the task, I will use critical thinking skills. Specifically, I will challenge my assumptions about the 'worst-case scenario' (fainting and going to the hospital and having them discover I have a disease). Wouldn't it be a good thing to discover it if something was actually wrong with my health? This would be a positive outcome of fainting because then they could treat the problem. Also, I will use grounding techniques to help me focus on the external environment instead of my body when I am forced to walk down the middle of the aisle.

you can use to cope when exposure tasks become difficult. Note that the time that it takes to complete the exposure tasks, as well as the time between each exposure task, will vary. It will depend on your specific tasks and your availability. My clients typically complete between two and five exposure tasks each week. Be sure to prioritize completing these tasks, however. It will be less effective if you let too much time pass between tasks.

Step 5: Let's do it! Get started on the exposure tasks you have decided to complete this week. Be sure to document all the details of your experience immediately after you complete your exposure task in the table below as well as to answer the reflection questions. This is a big part of the learning process. Good luck!

Table 10 Exposure experience log (with Ashonte's example)

Exposure task & date	Outcome & anxiety level (0–10)	Thoughts during exposure	Coping strategies used	Overall summary/ conclusion
Write the details of your task and date	Did you complete the task? What were your original predictions and fears? Did they come true? How was your anxiety? Were you able to cope with it?	What thoughts popped into your mind while completing the exposure?	What strategies did you use to cope with the anxiety during the exposure (e.g. challenging anxious thoughts, grounding exercises, coping cards)?	What are your overall conclusions from this task? Did you have any 'aha' moments or were any key lessons learned?
Drove five minutes to gas station alone (#5) Completed at 3pm on 12/23	I was able to complete the task. My biggest fear was that I would faint while driving. This did not happen. I made it safely to the store and back. I also predicted that I would experience a lot of fainting symptoms and would have to pull over but the symptoms were minimal and I was able to push through. Anxiety before task & in beginning (8/10) Anxiety toward the end of task (6.5/10)	At a few different points, I thought 'what if I faint?' And then images popped into my mind of my car crashing. My mind also kept drifting back to focus on my body to look for fainting signs.	I was able to challenge my anxious thoughts with Socratic questioning. When I started worrying that I would faint and crash, I reminded myself that this has never happened, despite all my fears. It helped a little bit. When I kept slipping up and hyper focusing on my body, I was able to redirect my attention to the external environment. My plan of using the audiobook really helped me with this.	It was scary at first and I almost didn't follow through with the task. But, overall, nothing bad happened other than being anxious and uncomfortable for a little bit. I also found that when I didn't give so much attention to my body and listened to my audiobook instead, I noticed fewer symptoms.

I shopped alone at a store for 15 minutes without using safety behaviors (#6) Completed on 10/25	I completed the task. My biggest fear was that I would faint in the store and there would be no one to help me (or someone would call an ambulance and I would be rushed to the hospital and find out terrible news). Neither of these things happened. I also thought the anxiety would be so overwhelming that I wouldn't be able to handle it. It wasn't as bad as I thought, however. Anxiety before task & into the middle (9/10) Anxiety toward the end (6/10)	I was very uncomfortable at first because I wasn't able to use any of my safety behaviors and this made me anxious. I slipped into the habit of focusing on my body to check for signs I might faint and kept thinking, 'oh no, I feel faint' or 'was that dizziness?' and at one point I catastrophized and thought, 'here we go, I am going to pass out.'	It really helped me to go back and question my feared scenarios—like, okay, if I faint what is the worst that can happen? I'll either just wake back up and I am sure people will help me get back up. Or, even if I go to the doctor, at least I am in good hands—like we had talked about before, if they find something wrong with me, well then it is good that I know now so I can do something about it. Also, it helped to use grounding techniques to help me re-focus on the external environment.	Although I felt really anxious at one point, it helped to realize that it wasn't the end of the world. I didn't like it. But nothing bad happened to me because I felt anxious. I was miserable for a few minutes but then it went away. Also, I ended up being okay, even without standing close to the side of the aisle, monitoring my body or bringing someone with me. No major events—no fainting and no going to the hospital and subsequently finding out terrible news.

Prior to getting started on your exposure exercises (as a part of Step 2), read through this list of tips to maximize learning during the exposure process.

Tips for designing an exposure hierarchy

- **Generalization:** When creating an exposure hierarchy, include a wide range of different activities as well as practice exposures in different settings. This can further solidify your learning because it allows you to continue to face fears and strengthen your skills, no matter the activity or setting. You can see an example of this in Ashonte's hierarchy. We exposed her to her fears while in a few different settings/activities (fear of fainting while driving, running, shopping). Generalization helps you learn you can face your fear anywhere.
- **Break up difficult tasks into smaller, manageable tasks:** For exposure tasks that are particularly difficult, you can split them into two or three separate tasks to slowly work your way up to the harder task. For example, Ashonte avoided going grocery shopping alone, driving or running because of her fear of fainting. We broke each of these types of exposures into two or three separate tasks. Specifically, we broke the task of shopping at a store into three tasks. This allowed Ashonte to start small and build her confidence as she slowly lengthened the task (i.e. shopping at a store and driving).
- **Slowly remove safety behaviors as you work your way up:** Although we want you to completely refrain from using any safety behaviors to maximize learning, if this is going to keep you from doing the exposure task, you can start small. In this case, slowly reduce the use of these behaviors as you build your confidence. Thus, connected to the tip above, you may allow yourself to use safety behaviors during the easier tasks at the bottom of the hierarchy. However, if you choose this option, keep in mind that you ultimately want to stop using safety behaviors all together. The items toward the top of the hierarchy should not permit the use of safety behaviors.
- **Be vivid and specific with your imaginal exposure tasks:** For imaginal exposures, you will write out the scenario and then will subsequently record it. When writing out the imaginal scenario,

make the details as vivid and specific as possible. This will help you connect with your story, making it more effective.

- **After completing your exposure hierarchy, you may want to design a new one:** Many times, after my client gets through their exposure hierarchy, we will design a new, refined hierarchy. This allows them to continue their practice of facing feared situations while refraining from safety behaviors. You may realize during your exposure tasks that particular situations you put yourself in were especially helpful. Thus, it may be helpful to include more challenging versions of that task in your new hierarchy, to allow you to continue to build your skills and confidence. This is why it is important to document all of your exposure experiences in your log so you can use this information to add and revise items in your next hierarchy.

Tips for completing tasks in exposure hierarchy

- **Prioritize your planning log:** Be sure to document your planned exposures in your planning log each week prior to completing the tasks (Table 12). Your planning log can be a helpful aid to ensure you answer important questions about your tasks prior to completing them. It is especially important to consider/document your predicted outcomes prior to engaging in the task. This will allow you to compare your predicted outcome with the actual outcome after the task is completed. Your planning log is also important to ensure that you anticipate and plan for challenges, stay organized and follow through with your tasks each week.
- **Try to accept and tolerate the anxiety during the exposure tasks:** Learn how to cope with anxiety instead of trying to get rid of it. One of the goals of exposure in general is to increase your distress tolerance skills. We want you to learn, through personal experience, that anxiety, while annoying, is safe and tolerable. We also want you to increase your sense of confidence and self-efficacy as you learn to trust in your ability to tolerate anxiety.
- **Use your adaptive coping techniques when exposure tasks get tough:** To help you successfully complete the exposure tasks, especially when they get uncomfortable or difficult to finish, use any of the adaptive coping skills you have acquired from this book or elsewhere. Some examples include:

- Challenging anxious thoughts with Socratic dialogue
- Coping cards (written reminders of the task purpose, words of encouragement)
- Attention training techniques to help you focus on the external environment
- Grounding exercises
- Controlled breathing exercises

- **Consider Socratic dialogue your best friend during exposures:** As mentioned in the tip above, Socratic dialogue should be a key resource to help get you through exposure tasks. Given this, I am providing a list of key questions you can ask yourself when you are either feeling hesitant to start the exposure task, start to become anxious during the task and/or find it difficult to get through the task. A few examples of some questions you can ask yourself during exposures:
  - What am I worried will happen during the exposure? Have I worried about this happening before and everything turns out to be okay?
  - In considering my feared outcome, can I explain *how* this would happen? Is this likely to happen? Is there another, more likely outcome?
  - If something negative does happen during the exposure, how could I respond and deal with it? What are some ways I (or others) would be able to manage the situation and cope with it? Could I envision the possibility that a negative outcome wouldn't be catastrophic?
  - If I am worried about anxiety symptoms, what specifically am I worried will happen? Has anxiety ever been dangerous for me? Can I learn to temporarily live with the discomfort of anxiety just like I have learned to deal with other unpleasant emotions (e.g. jealousy, anger, sadness)? In the past, has anxiety continued on ceaselessly or does it always dissipate over time?
- **Review imaginal exposures multiple times:** A helpful guideline with imaginal exposures is to listen to the recording multiple times. Ideally, you want to repeatedly listen to your recorded scenario until the anxiety you experience when listening to it (0–10) is cut down by about half (e.g. from 8/10 to 4/10).

- **Prioritize your exposure experience log:** Immediately after completing an exposure task, it is essential that you document everything in your exposure experience log (Table 13). This will solidify the learning process. Specifically, it can be useful to consider the difference between your predicted or feared outcomes and the actual outcome. More often than not, my clients realize that their feared outcome doesn't come true. Even in cases when there is a negative outcome or experience, they learn that they are able to cope with it much better than they assumed they would. In addition, it can be helpful to reflect on your exposure experience and draw your own conclusions from it.

Now that you have reviewed the tips, go back and complete the steps of developing and implementing your exposure hierarchy. My hope is that this experience will be empowering for you. Remember, these changes take time. Be diligent about completing your exposure tasks each week. The more you practice, the easier it will be to refrain from using these problematic behaviors. If it helps, enlist the support from an ally or trusted loved one who can hold you accountable for completing these tasks. Stick with it and you can rid yourself of these burdensome behaviors. Remember, change doesn't happen overnight. It happens by making small tweaks in your problematic behaviors each day.

Reference

1 Kemp JJ, Blakey SM, Wolitzky-Taylor KB, Sy JT, Deacon BJ. The effects of safety behavior availability versus utilization on inhibitory learning during exposure. *Cognitive Behaviour Therapy*. Published online February 14, 2019:1–12. <https://doi.org/10.1080/16506073.2019.1574312>

7

Live more comfortably with uncertainty

The intolerance of uncertainty, or IU, involves the interpretation of uncertain situations as being generally threatening and highly likely to produce negative outcomes.[1] In other words, if you can't be certain about a future thing, then that future thing is inevitably going to suck and you will be unable to deal with it. Research shows that people with health anxiety tend to be intolerant of any uncertainty when it comes to their health status.[2] Specifically, they often inaccurately assume that it is possible and necessary to be 100 percent certain that they won't experience a negative health outcome. Of course, we all know it is not possible to be certain about anything in the future and, unfortunately, health is no exception.

However, many health-anxious people have a difficult time accepting this. The reason for this is because people with high levels of IU tend to assume three things about uncertain situations.[1] Essentially, this whole process can paint a pretty grim picture of the future.

Table 1 Beliefs held by people with high intolerance of uncertainty

	Belief	Example
1	Uncertainty about a future thing probably means something bad is going to happen	A random headache for no identifiable reason probably means something is wrong
2	The bad thing in the future will probably be catastrophic	The headache is probably due to a brain tumor
3	I won't be able to deal with that very bad thing	I will be inconsolable. Doctors and medical resources won't be able to save me and I will die in three months

When a new symptom or bodily sensation emerges, many of my clients believe they must find the answer immediately or else they will be in serious trouble. In their minds, being unsure about the origin of a symptom is synonymous with danger. What's more, my clients often have a difficult time accepting explanations from doctors or results from tests. Thus, to deal with their fear of uncertainty when they can't find what they deem to be acceptable answers, they enter into a 'downward spiral' and engage in all sorts of unhelpful coping strategies, such as repeatedly seeking answers through doctors, tests, the internet and loved ones or excessively worrying about their health.[3,4]

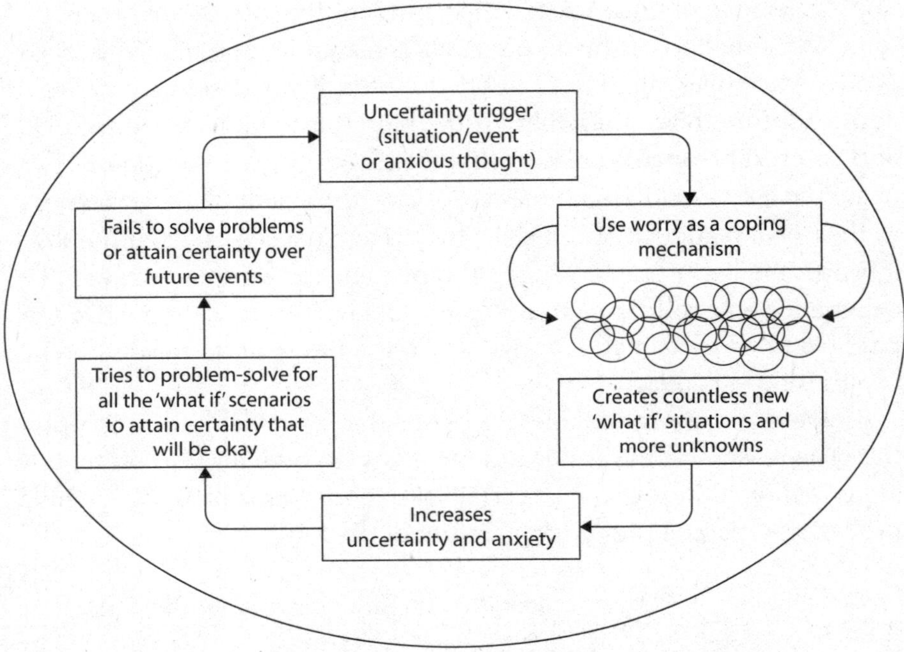

Unfortunately, these coping mechanisms only exacerbate the problem. As you know from the last chapter, safety behaviors such as reassurance-seeking foster dependence and further reinforce dysfunctional beliefs about health.

Although worry might *seem* productive, it is actually counterproductive. It gives you the *illusion* of certainty, as you might think it is preparing you for the worst so you will avoid any surprises. However, worry actually increases uncertainty. See, when people worry, they conjure up a variety of worst-case scenarios and then attempt to plan solutions for all the potential problems that arise in these terrible fictional scenarios. Given that this is all fiction, how many potential catastrophic outcomes are there? An infinite amount! So, essentially, worrying produces a bunch of distressing scenarios, which leads to more 'what if' questions and gives one even more reason to feel threatened by uncertainty.

Revising assumptions about uncertainty

If you struggle to tolerate uncertainty, there is hope. The overall goal is to learn to view uncertainty in new ways. Given that uncertainty in life is inevitable, we have to learn to live with it. But even if we could live in a certain world, it would undoubtedly be dull, boring and unfulfilling. It can be helpful to recognize and appreciate all of the beauty of living in an uncertain world. Not knowing what is going to happen tomorrow is what makes life interesting, exciting, adventurous, fun, beautiful. It also allows us to be challenged and promotes personal growth.[3]

More specifically, it is important that you learn to grow more comfortable with a *little* uncertainty when it comes to your health. Again, everyone struggles with uncertainty at times and that is okay. However, we want to help you get to a place in which you don't equate even the smallest amount of uncertainty with doom (e.g. assuming terrible things will happen just because you don't know the cause of every bodily change, sensation and symptom). This will help you refrain from futile (and exhausting) attempts to achieve absolute certainty about your health at all times.

Table 2 Growing comfortable with some uncertainty around health

	Belief	**Example**
1	Uncertain situations will probably turn out okay	This headache is probably due to something minor or benign.
2	Even if the symptom is due to something more serious, it probably won't be catastrophic.	If the headache is actually something more serious, it will most likely be treatable.
3	If I do face a health challenge or negative health outcome, I will be able to utilize personal, social and medical resources to cope.	I will have emotional and physical strength, social support and medical interventions to help me manage or cope with the illness.

The more you can tolerate uncertainty regarding your health, the less you will feel the desperate need to have control and, therefore, the less you will engage in the excessive worry and safety behaviors that are making you miserable. The goal of this chapter is to teach you cognitive and behavioral techniques that will help you view and respond to uncertainty differently.

The intolerance of uncertainty and thinking errors

When we believe that any amount of uncertainty about our health is inherently dangerous and unacceptable, this impacts how we interpret and respond to everything that happens in our daily life. Remember, our core beliefs guide what we pay attention to in our environment and how we interpret it.

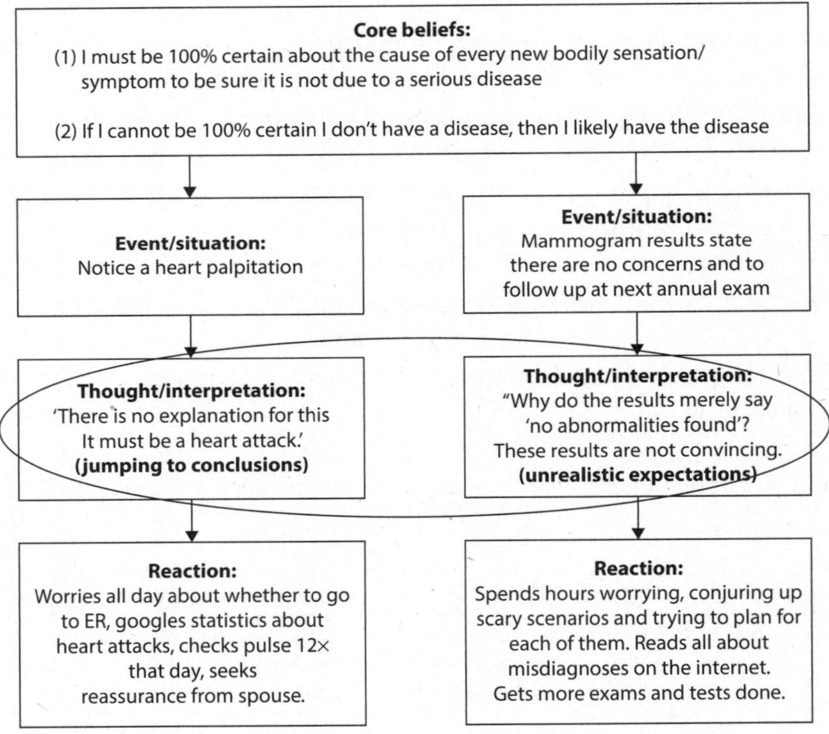

Core beliefs:
(1) I must be 100% certain about the cause of every new bodily sensation/symptom to be sure it is not due to a serious disease
(2) If I cannot be 100% certain I don't have a disease, then I likely have the disease
Event/situation:
Notice a heart palpitation
Event/situation:
Mammogram results state there are no concerns and to follow up at next annual exam
Thought/interpretation:
'There is no explanation for this It must be a heart attack.'
(jumping to conclusions)
Thought/interpretation:
"Why do the results merely say 'no abnormalities found'? These results are not convincing.
(unrealistic expectations)
Reaction:
Worries all day about whether to go to ER, googles statistics about heart attacks, checks pulse 12× that day, seeks reassurance from spouse.
Reaction:
Spends hours worrying, conjuring up scary scenarios and trying to plan for each of them. Reads all about misdiagnoses on the internet. Gets more exams and tests done.

For example, as you can see in this diagram, this core belief might lead you to have difficulty if you can't find a definitive explanation for every single bodily symptom or sensation. Or you might struggle when physicians, physical exams, labs or scans aren't able to provide answers with 100 percent certainty. You then engage in thinking errors and react in all sorts of unhelpful ways, making yourself miserable in the process. Below are a few examples of how the demand for certainty can lead one to think in distorted ways.

Unrealistic expectations: Experience difficulty when doctors and tests are unable to give you definitive answers or explanations for every potential question, concern or symptom/bodily sensation.

A high intolerance of uncertainty can result in unrealistic expectations, leading to distress when doctors or tests can't give enough assurance that everything is okay. My clients often are disappointed after receiving the results of a test or scan, even when they clearly indicate no cause for concern. In their mind, the results only confirm that the scan identified no abnormalities but did not mention anything about them being in good health. They expect that these tests should offer a certain degree of security and promise about their current or future health. I am not sure if they would be satisfied with anything short of the analyst including a little note at the bottom of the page to say, 'Don't worry, buddy! According to these results, you are in perfect health and will live well into your nineties.' However, such expectations are unrealistic, as it is not possible for a test, exam or anything else to offer that kind of certainty in life.

Yet, even when test results do provide some relief, it is short-lived, as eventually the uncertainty creeps back in again. My clients that tend to be 'care-seeking' would get tests done and would sometimes feel amazing immediately after receiving negative results. However, with every new passing hour, day, week after having received the results, this certainty faded. After all, they would rationalize that with the passing time came the possibility of something new developing in their body. The more days that stood between them and the test, the more they began to wonder again if they had something.

Jumping to conclusions: Interpreting the meaning of a health-related situation with little or no evidence. This can happen through mind reading or predicting health outcomes.

A high intolerance of uncertainty can also lead one to jump to conclusions when they are uncertain about the origin of bodily sensations or symptoms. My client, Olivia, frantically searched for answers when she noticed a mild rash on her leg, which was not accompanied by any other symptoms. She went to multiple doctors and had a few physical exams and tests done. Tests and exams revealed no concerns and doctors concluded it was likely due to something environmental (e.g. minor skin irritation, allergies, diet, weather, reaction to stress).

However, not knowing *exactly* what was causing the rash ate her alive. She hypothesized that the lack of a definitive conclusion about the rash's origin meant it really was something more serious that had not yet been identified, such as an autoimmune disease or cancer. She was consumed with worry, got more tests done and spent hours reading about the diseases she suspected were behind the symptom. Eventually, the rash went away and that specific fear faded. However, her desperate need to attain absolute certainty about the cause of the rash (instead of accepting that there was enough reason to believe it was not due to something serious) made her miserable for weeks.

> All-or-nothing thinking: Viewing health in absolute, black-and-white categories instead of taking a more balanced approach and seeing health and illness on a continuum.

When uncertainty is seen as dangerous and unacceptable, this can lead you to view health in rigid terms. My client, Sawyer, became highly anxious anytime she got sick, even if the sickness was relatively mild and common (e.g. a virus or cold). She worried that the mild sickness could either turn into something more serious if her immune system was weakened for some unknown reason or be inaccurately assumed to be a mild sickness when it was actually a serious disease.

Sawyer often rationalized that it was most likely a minor illness (given the symptoms and doctor's assessment). However, it was difficult for her to accept that there still was a *possibility* (no matter how slight) that the minor illness was due to an unidentified illness or could morph into something dangerous. Given this, she tended to see herself as being either healthy and 'safe' or sick and 'in danger.' She had a hard time seeing health as being on a spectrum or continuum and, instead, saw health as dichotomous.

Reconsider your view of uncertainty with cognitive techniques

The more you are able to tolerate a small amount of uncertainty when it comes to your health, the less you are going to worry about your health. What do I mean by this? I am not saying, *'Who cares, just don't think about your health and live for today... YOLO!'* Absolutely not. I am simply saying to learn to be okay with the fact that you can never know with 100 percent certainty that you won't have a negative health outcome. And you don't need to be 100 percent certain about your health to be safe. Just like you don't need to be 100 percent certain that you won't ever get into a fatal car accident to be safe. Yes, tragedy is possible. It happens, obviously. But it is not the most likely outcome. And, regardless, living in fear of negative or tragic circumstances robs you of the ability to enjoy the very life you are so intent on protecting. Learning to accept small amounts of uncertainty can be freeing.

Socratic dialogue to challenge the demand for certainty

One way to accomplish this is to evaluate and reconsider your assumptions. Specifically, we want to help you see that it is not possible to know the cause of every bodily sensation and symptom. Unless there is reason to be concerned (i.e. indicated by test/exam results, a doctor's concerns, persistence of symptoms) then it is likely due to normal benign bodily cues and sensations or minor conditions.

Further, we also want to help you recognize that not knowing with absolute certainty that you don't have a disease is not required in order for you to be safe, healthy and/or okay. Uncertainty does not equate to inevitable negative or catastrophic health outcomes. As you have done in other chapters, use the Socratic questions below to challenge any unhelpful assumptions about the need for certainty.

Socratic questions related to the intolerance of uncertainty

- How has the need for absolute certainty regarding my health made my life more difficult? How has this impacted my relationship with loved ones, finances, mental health, emotional well-being and life satisfaction?
- Are there any advantages to seeking certainty about my health? List them out and then take a closer look at each of them. Are there any advantages that may be not as advantageous as I am assuming? Can I take a moment to evaluate each of these perceived advantages and reframe any that might be more of a cost than an advantage?
- What could be some advantages of learning to accept a little uncertainty about my health? How might life be different and better if I learned to live more in the present moment instead of using worry to cope with the fear of uncertainty around my health?

- Do I tend to predict that something bad will happen with my health just because I am uncertain? Is it just as likely (or even more likely) that something good or neutral could happen when I am uncertain? What are some good/neutral outcomes of the uncertain situation?
- Am I assuming the *possibility* of having an illness means it is *probable* that I will have an illness?
- What is the likelihood that this uncertain situation will turn out to be catastrophic? If it is a small risk, can I live with this tiny chance? Can I, instead, focus on the more likely outcome?
- Do I tend to predict that something bad will happen with my health just because I am uncertain? Can I consider and list out some good or neutral outcomes that are more likely?
- When have uncertain or surprising circumstances or situations in my life turned out negative or bad in some way? How was I able to cope with this? What strengths do I have to help me cope with difficult situations in life?
- Have I ever faced uncertainty about my health and it turned out to be neutral, okay, or even positive? How often has this happened?
- If I have ever personally experienced a challenging health situation (or have witnessed a loved one experience a health challenge), how did I cope with the uncertainty around that health situation? Can I use that strength and apply those coping skills to any possible future situations?
- How many ways just this week have I accepted low or minimal risk in a variety of areas (e.g. driving to work or a friend's house, taking a flight, jogging outside on a busy street, swimming, using a knife to cut vegetables for dinner, using electrical appliances)?
- Is it possible that I am already skilled at accepting uncertainty in my life? In what ways in my daily life do I tolerate some uncertainty? What small risks am I okay with? Can I learn to take the same approach with my health—accept a little uncertainty because the risk is low?
- How do I view daily uncertainties in other areas of life? What do I do to deal with these uncertainties?
- How do other people I know cope with uncertainty in life or uncertainty about their health? What is their perspective? What strategies

do they use? Could I develop a similar outlook or use similar strategies when I am struggling to accept uncertainty with my health?

- What are the benefits of living in an uncertain world? For example, a pleasant surprise such as a surprise party, a baby, an engagement, an epiphany or discovery, a new career option?
- What unexpected but positive events have happened in my life (e.g. meeting a new friend/romantic interest unexpectedly, learning something new, receiving a gift, being suddenly inspired, making a career change)? How does all of this highlight the value of living in an uncertain, sometimes unpredictable world?
- Was there a time in my life when everything seemed to be unpredictable and uncertain? For example, as a child or adult did I ever experience adversity or trauma (e.g. abuse, neglect, poverty, violence, chaos/instability, illness in the family)? If so, through these experiences, did I (understandably) begin to assume that life, in general, is always unpredictable and even dangerous? Perhaps the assumptions I made and strategies I used to cope with all of this made sense at one time in my life. However, is it possible that assumptions and strategies are no longer necessary (or at least not to the same degree)?

Time to practice

Let's practice thinking about uncertainty in new ways. As you've been doing, review the list of common thinking errors below:

- All-or-nothing thinking
- Jumping to conclusions
- Catastrophizing
- Emotional reasoning
- Mental filter/Tunnel vision
- Unrealistic expectations
- Overgeneralization
- Magical thinking

I'd like you to start recognizing when you struggle to accept uncertainty in your daily life. For the next week, I want you to document in a thought record any thoughts that reflect this struggle. Any time you think you are having a hard time accepting even the smallest amount of uncertainty when it comes to your health, identify your thoughts and document the situation in your thought record. Next, challenge any thinking errors with the relevant Socratic questions above as well as any questions you come up with to critically evaluate and modify your assumptions.

Thought record to identify thinking errors and challenge thoughts

Date & situation or trigger & level of anxiety (1–10)

3/23

All test results (to assess for heart disease) came back normal a few months ago, but I still have random heart palpitations, fluttering and increased heart rate.

Anxiety: 9/10

Automatic thought about the situation & level of concern (1–10)

What if the test results were wrong? Or what if something has gone wrong with my heart in the last few months? It seems infeasible that these issues are just from anxiety—how do they know that for sure? If these test results are wrong, I could have a heart attack and die, leaving my kids without a mom. They won't be okay.

Level of concern: 9/10

Potential thinking errors

(1) Unrealistic expectations: expectations that these tests should be able to guarantee that I don't (or won't) have a heart problem, instead of accepting the results as most likely being accurate.

(2) Jumping to conclusions: making assumptions that my heart is in bad health based on a small amount of evidence (heart palpitations and increased heart rate) when there is more evidence to support the contrary (having three tests done with good results).

(3) Catastrophizing: assuming that even if there is (now or eventually) an issue with my heart, it automatically means heart attack, death and motherless children that will not be okay.

Response to thoughts or challenging with Socratic dialogue

It is highly unlikely that all of my test results are wrong. There is sound reason to believe that I am in good health and am very unlikely to have a heart attack. Just because it is possible that the test results are wrong (or I have a new issue that developed in the past couple of months) does not mean it is probable. I can learn to accept the small risk that the test is wrong just like I accept small, unlikely risks in so many other areas of life.

I am also jumping to conclusions and catastrophizing about a fairly normal and common bodily sensation that is also a common anxiety symptom. My doctors have recently ruled out any major concerns with my heart based on tests and have determined it to be anxiety. It is highly unlikely that they are wrong or that my heart health has changed dramatically since the tests were done a few months ago. I can live with the tiny possibility that there is an unidentified issue with my heart and can reassess at my next physical.

Living in a certain versus uncertain world

Imagine you wake up tomorrow morning and know every single detail about your day and exactly how you would experience it. You know exactly how breakfast would taste, the cute things your kids would say, the jokes your coworker would make, the praise you would receive from your supervisor, the angry insult from the guy in the car next to you while in traffic on the way home, the romantic surprise from your partner, the news that would hit the headlines, who would win the game and what you would dream about that night.

Now, imagine if you knew all of that detail about every single day for the rest of your life. How *boring* would that be? Uncertainty can be scary at times but it is also what makes life interesting, exciting, adventurous, fun and beautiful. Everything comes at a cost. It can be helpful to become more aware of the benefits of living in an uncertain world that are unique to you and your life.

To that end, instead of seeing uncertainty as inherently bad, work on recognizing its beauty. Perhaps you, like me, might conclude that there are many advantages to not knowing what is going to happen tomorrow. The reality is that in our beautiful, exciting and sometimes unpredictable world, we have to accept that good and bad things will occur. Instead of fearing and dreading the unknown, put your energy into enjoying the good and equip yourself to cope with the bad.

Try out a mental exercise. I want you to reflect for a few minutes about the times in your life when something unexpected turned out to be amazing. Perhaps it was meeting your partner, an epiphany, a surprise party, a promotion or new business venture, an experience while traveling, a brilliant idea, an unanticipated spiritual or religious transformation or welcoming a new child into your home. Consider that, if you lived in a certain world, you would lose all of the pleasure that comes with the positive unexpected surprises or life changes. I provide an example from my own life to help illustrate.

Table 3 Thought log of positive unexpected events

Unexpected event	What was it like to be surprised by this?	How did this add fulfillment to my life or change me?	How might my life be different if this unexpected event never took place?
While working toward my licensure hours after I got my master's degree, I unexpectedly had to switch clinical supervisors.	I was excited but also stressed because I didn't know how this would impact my timeline toward licensure.	My new clinical supervisor was both a therapist and a researcher in academia. We collaborated on a bunch of projects and I discovered a love for research. He is the reason I decided to go back and pursue a PhD.	Getting my PhD was one of the best decisions of my life. It changed my career trajectory in so many positive ways. I wouldn't be doing a lot of the things I am doing today if I didn't get my PhD.

Harnessing your existing skills

Although facing uncertainty about your health may seem overwhelming, you likely already have the ability to tolerate uncertainty in other areas without even realizing it. Think about the small risks you take every day, such as swimming, hiking, walking alone at night, eating in restaurants or jogging on a busy street. Many activities involve a tiny bit of risk in various ways but you accept the uncertainty that comes with it because the risk is small enough.

Every day I get into my car, there is a small chance I could get into a fatal car accident. I put preventative strategies in place, of course, to reduce this risk, such as driving safely and wearing a seatbelt. However, I have learned to accept that there is an unavoidable risk that, regardless of how carefully I drive, I *could* get into an accident. I accept this risk every day as I drive my family around Southern California. This is because I know that the benefits of driving (and, well, living life) outweigh the risks, given that the likelihood of a safe driver getting into a fatal accident is low enough.

It can be helpful to adopt a similar view when it comes to your health. Let's say you are someone with no major medical diagnoses. Every day you live your life not knowing *for sure* whether or not there is a disease developing in your body or you are on the verge of some major medical crisis. You can (and should) take *reasonable* steps to reduce the risk of this such as by getting your recommended screenings or seeking answers about symptoms as necessary. But beyond the reasonable steps, you can learn to live comfortably without the guarantee that you won't have a negative health outcome. Attaining certainty is not only an impossible goal but unnecessary. You can be safe (and certainly happy) without being 100 percent certain about whether you have a disease.

To shift your view, I invite you to recognize and harness the ability you already have to tolerate uncertainty in other areas of life so that you can learn to apply it to health-related situations. Think of it as having transferable skills. In what ways do you tolerate a little bit of uncertainty or risk in your day-to-day life? It might be helpful to think through your week. What activities do you engage in that pose a very small risk? In what ways have you learned to accept that you can't know the future? In what ways have you learned to accept that you can't guarantee you won't face serious psychological or physical harm?

Become more aware of the areas in which you are able to tolerate uncertainty by writing it down. Then, you can borrow from this skill set when you face uncertainty related to your health. Importantly, this exercise is not intended to encourage you to ruminate on everything that could go wrong in other areas of your life. Remember, you tolerate uncertainty and take small risks in other areas of your life for *good reason*, because the risk is low. This is adaptive. We are recognizing your ability to do this because we want you to apply this adaptive skill to your health. To illustrate, I'll offer a few examples from my own life.

Table 4 My record of how I tolerate small amounts of uncertainty or low risk

Action/Situation	Uncertainty/Potential risk
Hiking in Griffith Park	I could get bit by a rattlesnake.
Sending my kids to school	They could be bullied, kidnapped or shot.
Jogging on a sidewalk	A drunk driver could swerve and run me over.
Trusting my husband	He could cheat on me.
Taking a bath alone	I could randomly faint and drown.
Driving on the freeway	I could get into a fatal car accident.
Trusting close friends with the private, embarrassing details of my life	They could tell people things that would embarrass me and I would be really hurt.
Driving on a bridge	I could get into a crash and slide off the bridge.
Eating sashimi	I could get really sick from being exposed to a parasite, virus or bacteria.
Swimming in the ocean	I could get caught in an undercurrent and drown.

Think through why you are able to tolerate these small risks every day. In my case, I know that everything listed in my log is highly unlikely and some of them are so unlikely that they are nearly impossible. I also know that I have and can continue to take protective measures in all of these categories to further reduce any risk (e.g. being in a relationship with people who have demonstrated trustworthiness, talking to my children about bullying, practicing safe driving, heeding warnings regarding ocean safety). Lastly, I know that, even in the rare chance (or in some of these cases, *very rare*) that any of these bad things do happen, there are actions that can be taken to help me cope or deal with it.

Behavioral techniques to help you tolerate uncertainty

You've learned how to use cognitive techniques to reshape how you see uncertainty. Now, you will learn a couple of behavioral techniques to help you better cope with uncertainty. Specifically, we will use mindfulness strategies to help you gain a sense of control over your worry and focus on the present moment. We will also use an experiment to allow you to test your assumptions about uncertainty and reduce your fear of it. These exercises can help you get more comfortable with uncertainty and become less reliant on counterproductive coping strategies.

Mindfulness of worry thoughts

When we struggle with uncertainty about our health, we fall into the trap of engaging in excessive worry as a maladaptive coping strategy. For example, if we can't be certain about the cause of a new bodily sensation, we might frantically look for information and then try to think through all of the 'what ifs' so we can problem-solve and gain a greater sense of certainty. However, as you know by now, this is counterproductive, as worry only produces more worry thoughts, creating even more uncertainty.

One strategy to reduce the use of worry as a coping strategy is mindfulness of worry thoughts. Mindfulness is the practice of being more aware of your present-moment experiences and surroundings with an attitude that is open, flexible, curious, accepting and non-judgmental.[4,5] By its very nature, mindfulness is the antithesis of worry. The key components of mindfulness are the opposite of the key components of worry, with its focus on future events and rigid, non-acceptance of uncertainty. This is why mindfulness is a common intervention used to treat Generalized Anxiety Disorder, a disorder for which excessive worry is the most salient feature.[6] In general, people with anxiety will be more likely to thrive the closer they can stay to the present moment.

Mindfulness training can involve many different strategies, depending on the needs and goals of the individual. Using mindfulness to disengage with worry involves reshaping how you see the worry thoughts you have and changing your relationship with them. We don't simply want to tell you to disengage with your worry thoughts because, well, it's not helpful to hear that if you haven't tried it before. We want you to test out the *experience* of disengaging with your worry thoughts.

Essentially, we want you to practice seeing your thoughts as passing mental events instead of viewing them as facts. Notice them, sure, but don't give them too much of your attention or focus. Let them pass on by. You don't need to suppress them but you also don't need to better understand them or take them too seriously. Try to stay somewhere near the middle of this diagram.

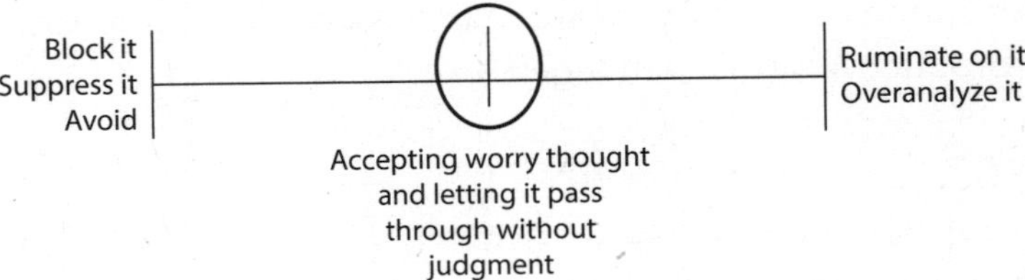

Five-minute exercise: Practicing mindfulness of worry thoughts

To practice mindfulness of worry thoughts, we will need to do what is sometimes referred to as a 'worry induction' or 'worry exposure.' This means we will have you intentionally bring a distressing worry thought to the forefront of your mind. We will then be able to use that worry as a tool to help you practice disengagement from it. Essentially, we want you to practice experiencing the worry and then subsequently disengage from it.

1 Set a timer, close your eyes and think of something you have recently worried about. Spend a few moments thinking about that worry. Sit with it for a moment. Rate your anxiety level on a scale from 0–10, 10 being the highest level of anxiety. It is ideal if your anxiety at the beginning of this exercise is relatively high, I'd say around a 7 or higher. We want the worry thought to be distressing enough that it is comparable to the worry you might have in your regular daily experience. This will help you build confidence in your ability to use this skill when you face typical worries in your daily life.
2 Keep your eyes closed and, after you've sat with that worry thought for a little bit, pivot and take notice of your breathing. Pay attention to your breath as it flows in and out of your body. Notice how your chest, lungs and stomach feel as they expand and contract. Notice any tension or release in your body. You do not need to alter your breathing patterns in any way. Simply observe them.
3 As you are observing your breathing patterns, your worry may fight its way back into your mind. Or your mind might wander to other thoughts. That's okay. Don't judge or criticize yourself for it. Just notice that it happened and gently redirect your focus back to the details of your breathing patterns. You will likely notice that thoughts will sporadically pop into your mind throughout this exercise. This is what our minds do. Each time it happens, simply normalize it and accept it. And then shift your focus back to the sensations of breathing. Don't push the thought away. Don't hold onto it. Don't

analyze it. Simply notice and pivot back to breathing. At the end of five minutes, open your eyes.

Let's discuss. Using a mindfulness exercise is one way to gain a sense of control over the worry by disengaging from it. Remember, when we feel uncertain about something, we tend to worry as a coping strategy. We might assume that the worry process is helping us by getting us closer to certainty. However, worry only fuels more worry thoughts, which creates even more uncertainty. You essentially enter a 'worry loop,' which can be hard to break away from. Once you have learned how to disengage and focus on something else, you can continue to practice this skill. Like with anything, the more you practice this the better you will get at it.

It's time to reflect! It can be helpful to document the details of your mindfulness experience in the log below (see the example). Like other exercises we have completed, reflection allows you to focus on some of the important lessons and further reinforces learning. I recommend doing this exercise for five minutes every day for a week. Over time, you can increase the length of the exercise (e.g. 10 minutes, 15 minutes) to continue building this skill.

Table 5 Mindfulness reflection log

Date of exercise & length of exercise	Worry thought for worry induction (& anxiety rating in the beginning 0–10)	How was the experience? Were you able to recognize when the worry popped up? Were you able to let it go and redirect? Did having a different, neutral focal point (i.e. your breath) help take your focus away from the worry at all?	Anxiety rating at the end (0–10)
Monday/ Five minutes	I worried that the new mole I noticed this week was some type of cancer. Anxiety level: 7/10	It was hard at first because I felt anxious once I started thinking about the mole. Every time I focused on my breathing, my mind quickly returned to the mole. And then other thoughts crept in. But it helped to think of it as not a big deal and that it is normal to mentally drift. Once I got in the habit of simply redirecting back to my breathing, it got a little easier. It did help to have something else to turn my focus to. I think with more practice, I'll get better.	3.5/10

The 'Waiting' experiment

As we've discussed, people with health anxiety tend to assume that uncertainty equals danger. For example, you might assume that if you don't know the origin of the symptom, it must be serious and could potentially be catastrophic. And, sure, it is possible that a random symptom you are having is due to something serious. But a random symptom is much more likely to be due to random body noise or a non-catastrophic illness. However, the uncertainty of it all can seem like it is eating you alive. Because *what if* it is actually due to something really serious? It doesn't matter how tiny the chance is when there is still a chance. Indeed, the 'what if' game is all about uncertainty.

Let's say you are someone who gets car sick easily. You take a drive up the mountains with some friends for a ski trip and after circling your way up the mountain for a few minutes, you start feeling nauseous. This situation doesn't puzzle you because you've been here before, many times. On windy roads, you get car sick. Mystery solved. But what if you randomly started feeling nauseous while at home working on your computer? The origin of this symptom is not so obvious. In fact, it might be a completely new experience. Not knowing where this symptom is coming from means *anything* is possible. And that anything could be catastrophic. Hence, you enter the ever familiar downward spiral of thinking errors and problematic behaviors, all in the effort to reduce the uncertainty of the situation.

But what if you could learn to sit with the uncertainty, just for a little bit? I often have my clients try the 'waiting experiment' to help them get more comfortable with uncertainty. The 'waiting experiment' is a behavioral strategy that involves waiting for a brief period of time before rushing to seek answers about a mild symptom or bodily sensation (e.g. 3 days, 1 week, 2 weeks). At the end of the waiting period, if the symptom is still present and is bothering them, they can (and do) take steps to address it, which often includes going to the doctor.

This exercise can help you practice tolerating the discomfort of uncertainty. It is also often used to help one refrain from the use of safety behaviors, which we focused on in the last chapter. We will use it to help you work toward both goals: (1) build your tolerance of uncertainty; and (2) continue the work we did in Chapter 6 on refraining from the use of safety behaviors.

Preparing for the 'Waiting' experiment

Let's experiment. The next time you have a minor symptom or bodily sensation, refrain from drawing conclusions about the symptom, checking it excessively or seeking reassurance from loved ones, the internet or the doctor for three days. During this time period, you will likely notice an increase in your sense of uncertainty about the symptom. This is expected of course, given that you are not allowing yourself to do any of the things you normally do to seek certainty about what is causing the symptom. Try to think of the increase in uncertainty during this experiment as a benefit. It is allowing you to practice the skill of tolerating uncertainty and anxiety.

Before doing the experiment, consider: *What do you predict will happen if you wait three days before going to the doctor?* Write down your predictions. For example, your predictions might include:

Prediction 1: I won't be able to handle/manage the anxiety and discomfort of being uncertain about what is causing the symptom. It will overwhelm me.

Prediction 2: This symptom could be something serious and will be deadly if I don't address it right away.

It is important to consider what you predict or expect to happen prior to engaging in any experiment. These predictions are what we will be testing. The goal is to help you learn that: (1) you can tolerate the anxiety and uncertainty (and even if you struggle to tolerate it in the beginning, practice will help you improve this skill over time); and (2) your predictions about what will happen when you are uncertain about a symptom are often inaccurate (and even if not, you can likely cope better than you assume you can).

Gathering the results of the experiment

During the three-day waiting period, monitor your thoughts and anxiety level in a thought log. This can help you learn to see the patterns in your thoughts and anxiety over the three-day period. *In the spirit of improving your tolerance of uncertainty, I want you to pay special attention to any thoughts related to this struggle.* Again, during this waiting period, you will notice a heightened sense of uncertainty, which will likely make you feel more anxious.

Therefore, you will want to use techniques to help you when you feel particularly anxious. You can use the mindfulness exercises we just discussed (or the attention redirection exercises in Chapter 5) to help you turn your focus away from your worries if the experiment becomes challenging at times. Most importantly, similar to when you completed exposure tasks in Chapter 6, I want you to use your cognitive restructuring skills to help you cope with anxious moments during this experiment. You can draw from the questions in Table 1 or from the list below.

A few Socratic questions that might be helpful if the uncertainty/ anxiety is heightened during the experiment:

- What am I worried will happen during the experiment? Have I worried about this happening before and everything turns out okay?
- If the symptom does worsen or doesn't go away during the three-day period, how can I deal with it? What actionable steps can I plan to take in that case?
- If I am struggling with anxiety and uncertainty during the experiment, how can I cope? Can I use mindfulness strategies or other adaptive coping skills, such as engaging in pleasant activities or hobbies?
- If I am worried about anxiety symptoms, what specifically am I worried will happen? Has anxiety ever been dangerous for me? Can I consider that discomfort (e.g. anxiety) is not fun but it is not dangerous? Have I learned to live with other unpleasant emotions (e.g. jealousy, anger, sadness)? How might learning to live with a little bit of discomfort help me in this situation as well as in future situations?

Experiment reflection

After you have completed the experiment, it is critical to evaluate the results and your experience. Try not to skip this part because the conclusions you draw from this will likely influence future situations. Specifically, if you are able to learn that your predicted outcomes were different from the actual outcomes, this can serve as a reminder the next time you find yourself desperately wanting to seek certainty. Or,

Table 6 The waiting experiment experience log (Friday at 4pm–Mon at 4pm)

Symptom of concern: Small bump on scalp				
Day/time	**Thoughts about symptom**	**Level of anxiety and uncertainty (0–10)**	**Any impulse to seek certainty (e.g. through excessive worry, safety behaviors)?**	**Were you able to withstand the impulse to seek certainty? How so?**
Friday at 4pm	What if this is cancer? I shouldn't have agreed to this.	9/10	Yes—I hate not knowing and want to go to urgent care right away. I also am having a hard time not slipping into the old patterns of worrying about the symptom.	Yes—I challenged my catastrophic thoughts and reminded myself I can go to the doctor in a couple of days if necessary.
Friday at 7pm	What if this is an infection of some kind? It will be much worse, possibly fatal, by the time I go to the doctor.	10/10	Yes—I am feeling even more anxious than before. Maybe I should go to the ER? I keep worrying, as I mentally replay 'what if' scenarios about this symptom.	Yes—again I challenged my thoughts. I considered the fact that I still don't have any other symptoms, other than the bump (and if it was an infection or something dire I would likely have other symptoms).
Saturday at 1pm	The bump is still there. But if it is serious, I am sure I will be fine for the next day until I go to the doctor. I will find out and can deal with it.	8/10	I don't feel as strong of an urge to go to the doctor or seek answers. But I still feel a little bit anxious about not knowing what is causing this bump.	Yes—I didn't have as much of an impulse. Anytime I started to think about it, I just reminded myself I can go to the doctor soon if necessary.
Sunday at 2pm	The bump seems smaller. Maybe it is nothing.	6/10	I am feeling a lot better. The bump is smaller and I am starting to wonder if it wasn't a big deal after all.	Yes—I was able to refrain from seeking certainty. The anxiety improved a lot.
Monday at 10am	I can barely feel the bump. I think it might be a pimple.	4/10	I am a lot less anxious. It helps that the bump is smaller. But I think I got just a little more comfortable with not knowing for sure.	Yes. I'm still going to make a doctor appointment at the end of the 3 days. But I have very little anxiety.

even if you had a negative experience during this experiment (i.e. the anxiety and uncertainty did feel overwhelming), you still might have gained some insight into how to cope.

After you complete this exercise, try to spend at least ten minutes answering a few questions about your experiment experience:

- Were you able to hold off on engaging in excessive worry and your safety behaviors and live with the uncertainty for the specified time?
- Was the anxiety or uncertainty unbearable or were you able to manage it? Did it improve over time?
- How did you cope with the anxiety and uncertainty?
- What was the outcome? Was the symptom a sign of a serious disease? Was it benign body noise or a minor illness? Or did it go away all together?
- Did you end up going to the doctor or seeking information about the symptom after the three-day waiting period? What was the outcome?
- What might be your conclusions about this experience?

Remember, the goal of this experiment is to (1) practice tolerating anxiety and uncertainty as well as to (2) refrain from unhelpful behaviors when you are uncertain about a symptom. I would suggest using this experiment periodically to help you continue building your tolerance of uncertainty as well as to help you continue to reduce your use of safety behaviors.

I still use this practice today. If I notice a new random symptom, such as a rash, I challenge myself to wait a few days before I potentially overreact. Again, you can also do this experiment for a longer period of time (e.g. 1 or 2 weeks). Sometimes, I do go to the doctor after the waiting period is over because the symptom is still there or has worsened and/or additional symptoms have emerged. However, there have been plenty of times that the symptom was just random body noise and is completely gone by the third day. In sum, this experiment helps me to not assume that *every* unexplained bodily sensation is a catastrophe.

References

1 Dugas M, Robichaud M. *Cognitive-Behavioral Treatment for Generalized Anxiety Disorder: From Science to Practice.* Routledge; 2007.

2 Fetzner MG, Asmundson GJG, Carey C, et al. How do elements of a reduced capacity to withstand uncertainty relate to the severity of health anxiety? *Cognitive Behaviour Therapy*. 2014;43(3):262–274. <https://doi.org/10.1080/16506073.2014.929170>

3 Fergus TA. Cyberchondria and intolerance of uncertainty: Examining when individuals experience health anxiety in response to internet searches for medical information. *Cyberpsychology, Behavior, and Social Networking.* 2013;16(10):735–739. <https://doi.org/10.1089/cyber.2012.0671>

4 Horenstein A, Rogers AH, Bakhshaie J, Zvolensky MJ, Heimberg RG. Examining the role of anxiety sensitivity and intolerance of uncertainty in the relationship between health anxiety and likelihood of medical care utilization. *Cognitive Therapy and Research*. 2018;43(1):55–65. <https://doi.org/10.1007/s10608-018-9980-z>

5 Keng SL, Smoski MJ, Robins CJ. Effects of mindfulness on psychological health: a review of empirical studies. *Clinical Psychology Review*. 2011;31(6):1041–1056. doi:https://doi.org/10.1016/j.cpr.2011.04.006

6 American Psychiatric Association. Diagnostic and statistical manual of mental disorders. *Diagnostic and Statistical Manual of Mental Disorders*. 2013;5(5). doi:https://doi.org/10.1176/appi.books.9780890425596

8

Find a little hope in medical resources

People with health anxiety tend to view the field of medicine as wholly insufficient and incapable.[1] In other words, many people with severe health anxiety assume, or fear, that medical providers, tests and treatments will be unable to help them identify and treat a disease. This can play out in many ways. After a medical appointment or receiving the results of an assessment or test, one might doubt a doctor's assessment or the validity of a test. They also might struggle when medical providers, assessments and tests aren't able to give them definitive answers with 100 percent accuracy (note that the intolerance of uncertainty plays a role in this as well). Or they might believe that getting a disease is synonymous with death because they assume medical providers or interventions won't be able to help them manage or overcome the disease. All of this can make a health-anxious person feel doubtful, dissatisfied, suspicious and more anxious while interacting with the healthcare system.

To take adequate care of our bodies and optimize our health, we need to engage in health-promoting behaviors, such as getting the recommended physicals and screenings, consulting about new symptoms as necessary and treating disease. Thus, it is important to revise beliefs that might interfere with our ability to have a functional, adaptive relationship with healthcare and those that provide it. It is not within the scope of this book to discuss the many flaws of the healthcare system in the United States (e.g. insurmountable cost of healthcare services and prescription drugs, restrictions and limitations imposed by insurance companies, overworked medical providers, discrimination, focus on reactionary care instead of preventative care, to name just a few examples). Even if you are outside of the USA, I am sure you too suffer repercussions from the flaws in your own healthcare system.

Nonetheless, despite the barriers we face, it is in our best interest to identify more helpful ways of viewing and engaging with medical providers and interventions for the sake of both our physical and mental health. Specifically, we want to help you to increase your sense of self-efficacy to advocate for yourself as well as to develop a *reasonable* amount of trust in the competency and capability of medical providers, tests and treatment options. Doing this will help you become less fearful of disease because you will be able to assume, at least on some level, that a medical condition can be adequately detected and managed.

My client, Alma, worried about getting a late-stage cancer diagnosis. She feared that doctors and tests wouldn't accurately detect the cancer until it was 'too late' and the disease was too advanced to be effectively treated. This fear led Alma to check her body regularly so that she could aid medical providers in identifying any early signs of cancer. She also frequently went to the doctor, switching primary care doctors and specialists if they didn't find anything or weren't able to explain symptoms that she perceived to be a sign of cancer. As a result of all of this, she spent an exorbitant amount of money on excessive medical appointments and repeatedly getting scans, bloodwork and assessments done. This diagram illustrates how Alma's behavior impacted her daily life.

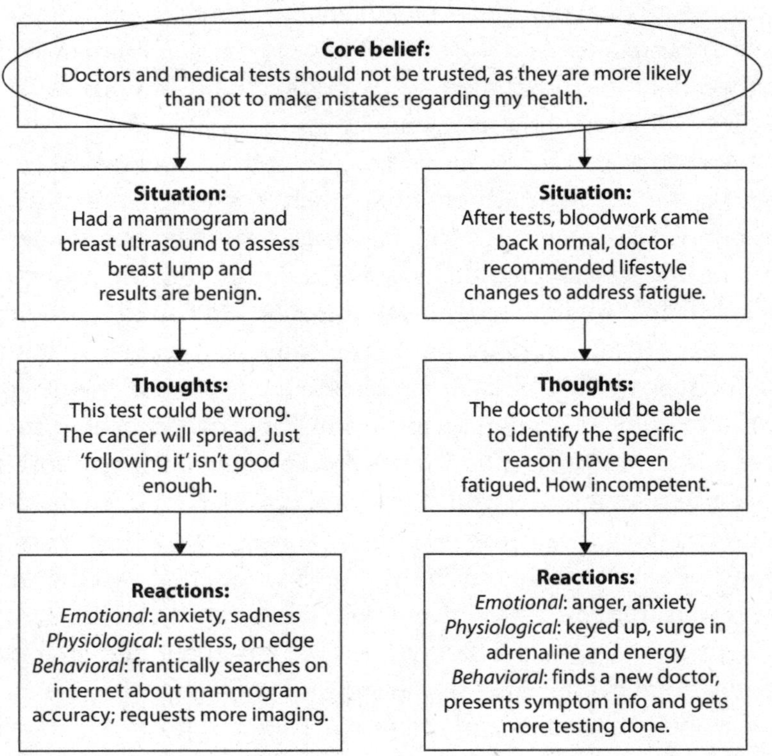

Core belief:
Doctors and medical tests should not be trusted, as they are more likely than not to make mistakes regarding my health.
Situation:
Had a mammogram and breast ultrasound to assess breast lump and results are benign.
Thoughts:
This test could be wrong. The cancer will spread. Just 'following it' isn't good enough.
Reactions:
Emotional: anxiety, sadness
Physiological: restless, on edge
Behavioral: frantically searches on internet about mammogram accuracy; requests more imaging.
Situation:
After tests, bloodwork came back normal, doctor recommended lifestyle changes to address fatigue.
Thoughts:
The doctor should be able to identify the specific reason I have been fatigued. How incompetent.
Reactions:
Emotional: anger, anxiety
Physiological: keyed up, surge in adrenaline and energy
Behavioral: finds a new doctor, presents symptom info and gets more testing done.

It is important to acknowledge that Alma's fear of having an unidentified or misdiagnosed health issue is valid in that it can happen. You might even have experienced this or know someone who has, which we will dive into in a minute. And part of taking care of ourselves is being aware, to a reasonable degree, of what is going on with our bodies and seeking answers for health concerns. However, we move into the territory of dysfunctional thinking and behavior when we assume these situations are likely or inevitable. To that end, these problematic assumptions and behaviors are what Alma and I targeted in treatment.

Medical trauma or medical adversity

Core beliefs develop initially from significant life experiences, as we have discussed throughout this book. There are many who have faced one particular type of life experience that may have altered their view of medical care and, ultimately, increased their health anxiety: *medical trauma or medical adversity. Medical trauma* is a range of psychological and physiological reactions to injury, pain, serious disease, medical procedures and invasive or distressing treatment experiences.[2,3] It can occur as a result of a medical crisis, receiving a life-altering or life-threatening medical diagnosis, having problematic or frightening experiences during interactions with providers or during the diagnostic or treatment process.[4]

Some experiences may be adverse but not necessarily traumatic. For example, you may have had challenging experiences in the medical setting that didn't traumatize you, per se, but have still impacted your sense of safety, trust and power when it comes to interacting with the medical setting. Regardless, challenging experiences in the medical setting can be frightening, disorienting and disempowering and, in their more extreme form, can lead to:[4]

- post-traumatic stress
- anxiety
- depression
- substance abuse
- other secondary crises.

And, since engaging with the medical setting is necessary to take care of our bodies, addressing any relevant mental barriers is warranted.

Perhaps you have personally experienced adversity or trauma in the medical setting. Maybe you know loved ones who have experienced this or have witnessed people experience this as a caregiver or medical provider. Or perhaps you have simply heard about these types of situations and fear that it will happen to you. Regardless, it is necessary to dissect your experiences or fears and recognize their impact and how they have shaped your beliefs about getting medical care and your overall health.

Casey

My client, Casey, was experiencing chronic pain that resulted from a shoulder injury. She was told it would improve over time, but instead the pain worsened. After several months, she started experiencing symptoms of depression because the pain was limiting her ability to engage in the usual activities that brought her joy, including weight lifting, rock climbing and tennis. She also noticed an increase in anxiety because she felt helpless and like she had lost control of her life in many ways.

She saw her doctor several times, who told her that the physical pain was likely being exacerbated by her depression and anxiety. He believed that once they found the right psychiatric medication and got her psychiatric symptoms under control, the pain would dissipate. After a couple of years with no improvement, she switched doctors and got a second opinion. It turned out that her injury was not healing as it should. After several medical interventions, including a surgery, the pain finally improved. Of course, as her life got back to normal and she was able to enjoy activities again, her depression also improved.

However, not surprisingly, this experience triggered Casey's health anxiety. She began to worry about her health often and became hypervigilant about every bodily sensation. She spent a lot of time googling symptoms and diseases or injuries. Also, her negative experiences with her first doctor led her to avoid interactions with medical providers as much as possible.

When we started to dig deeper into her fears, we realized her newfound focus on her body was because she had lost the ability to trust in doctors, tests and treatments. After years of her issue being dismissed and incorrectly diagnosed, she believed that *any* future health problem would likely also go unaddressed and she would inevitably suffer. Therefore, she decided she needed to start taking matters into her own hands, so to speak.

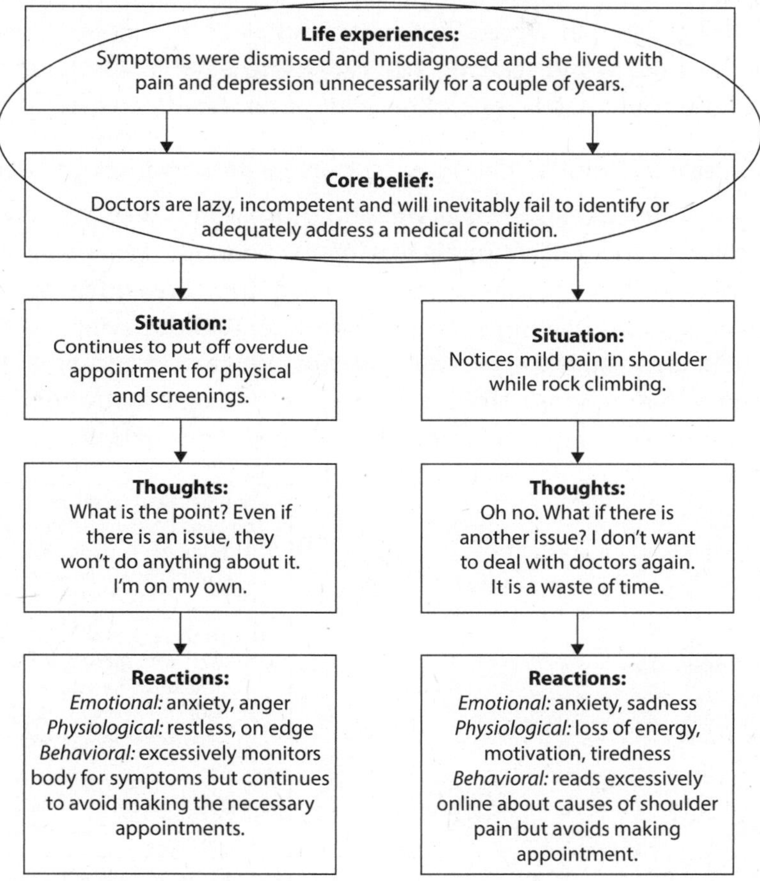

Life experiences:
Symptoms were dismissed and misdiagnosed and she lived with pain and depression unnecessarily for a couple of years.
Core belief:
Doctors are lazy, incompetent and will inevitably fail to identify or adequately address a medical condition.
Situation:
Continues to put off overdue appointment for physical and screenings.
Situation:
Notices mild pain in shoulder while rock climbing.
Thoughts:
What is the point? Even if there is an issue, they won't do anything about it. I'm on my own.
Thoughts:
Oh no. What if there is another issue? I don't want to deal with doctors again. It is a waste of time.
Reactions:
Emotional: anxiety, anger
Physiological: restless, on edge
Behavioral: excessively monitors body for symptoms but continues to avoid making the necessary appointments.
Reactions:
Emotional: anxiety, sadness
Physiological: loss of energy, motivation, tiredness
Behavioral: reads excessively online about causes of shoulder pain but avoids making appointment.

Casey's experience with her first doctor was awful and her subsequent doubt and mistrust were understandable. The problem, however, was that the doubt and mistrust led her to develop debilitating anxiety about her health and avoid medical care, which over time can have a significant negative impact on her health. Avoidance of trauma-related stimuli is a common coping mechanism among those who experience *all* types of trauma.[5] However, this poses a unique type of challenge for those with medical trauma, given that going to medical settings, and possibly facing trauma-related stimuli, is a necessary part of taking care of one's body (particularly when one has a medical condition). Despite this, some research shows that people often avoid medical settings in the aftermath of traumatic or negative experiences in health care.[4,6] One of our treatment goals was to help Casey modify some of her beliefs and behaviors so that she could rebuild a small or *reasonable* amount of trust in healthcare and seek medical care as necessary. Reshaping beliefs and behaviors ultimately helped her reduce her health anxiety.

Dysfunctional beliefs give way to biased information processing

When we hold a belief, we seek out and process information in a way that reinforces that belief. This is true of any adaptive or maladaptive belief we have. But you can imagine the negative consequences of a maladaptive belief gaining strength over time. Without even realizing it, we feed these beliefs every day with how we take in and process everything that happens around us. And, of course, the stronger the belief, the more it is going to negatively impact your daily life.

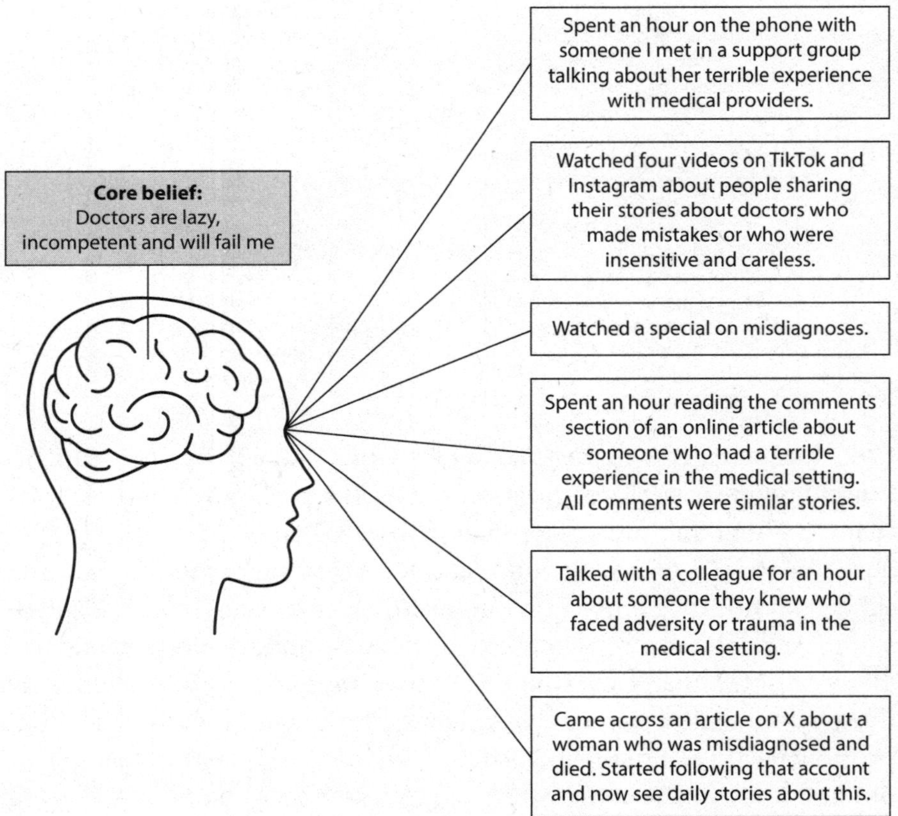

Core belief:
Doctors are lazy, incompetent and will fail me
Spent an hour on the phone with someone I met in a support group talking about her terrible experience with medical providers.
Watched four videos on TikTok and Instagram about people sharing their stories about doctors who made mistakes or who were insensitive and careless.
Watched a special on misdiagnoses.
Spent an hour reading the comments section of an online article about someone who had a terrible experience in the medical setting. All comments were similar stories.
Talked with a colleague for an hour about someone they knew who faced adversity or trauma in the medical setting.
Came across an article on X about a woman who was misdiagnosed and died. Started following that account and now see daily stories about this.

Let's look at how Casey's belief is strengthened by her selective attention and information processing, as illustrated in the diagram above. First, Casey's frightening, disempowering and frustrating experience led her to believe that, in general, doctors and other medical providers are lazy and incompetent. Having had these experiences and now holding these beliefs, she is quick to notice other similar situations or stories. Casey joins a support group for managing the challenges around injuries/ medical issues (a good thing) and in this group discovers that a couple of others have had negative experiences in the medical setting. She also reads stories about this in online forums and articles and watches videos on social media. Of course, online algorithms for news feeds and social media platforms curate what we see based on viewing history and, thus, exponentially magnify this process.

Through all of these activities, Casey reasoned negative experiences in the medical setting are inevitable and automatically catastrophic. Eventually, any positive story about someone receiving adequate or good medical care seemed like the rare exception. And, of course, as these beliefs grew stronger, so did the problematic thoughts and behaviors in her daily life. In treatment, I helped Casey intentionally modify the environmental stimuli she consumed as well as how she processed this information. This helped her to alter her beliefs over time.

Revising perspectives and rebuilding trust and hope

Alma's and Casey's situations illustrate a key point: the fear of having a current or future health issue that goes unidentified, misdiagnosed or ineffectively treated is very common among those who live with health anxiety. This can certainly be true if you have experienced any kind of medical trauma but it can also be a salient fear even if you have not directly experienced medical trauma. After all, these unfortunate, difficult and sometimes tragic situations do happen. And if it is possible, then there is always the lingering question of: *what if* this happens to me or *what if* this happens to me again? The problem is this 'what if' question begins to rule your life.

The goal, therefore, is to learn how to revise thoughts, beliefs and behaviors so that you don't have to live in fear of this 'what if' question. Note that the goal is *not* to convince you to have blind trust in medical providers or interventions. Obtaining a second opinion and/or switching doctors is certainly necessary at times, as you can see in Casey's situation. However, it can become problematic if you are continually seeking out second, third or fourth opinions (what we often refer to as 'doctor shopping') or if you tend to make sweeping overgeneralizations about the inadequacy or insufficiency of the medical field. We want to revise thinking and behavior that demonstrate a general *pattern* of mistrust, skepticism and doubt.

The cost–benefit analysis

For those who believe that medical providers, tests and treatments are overall incapable and untrustworthy, an important question is: just how much does this belief impact your life? We last discussed this in Chapter 6 when we explored the costs and benefits of safety and avoidance behaviors, but we can use the same strategy to explore the impact of problematic beliefs too. This strategy can help you see just how much the beliefs about the field of medicine are helping you or hurting you. See page 132 in Chapter 6 to review a detailed breakdown of why this strategy is helpful and how to implement it, step by step.

Tony

Tony, a former client, had severe health anxiety. Like many other people with health anxiety, he held a lot of unhelpful and maladaptive beliefs about health, including the belief that doctors and tests are generally incompetent and incapable. His cousin had a late-stage cancer diagnosis, and she had to undergo chemo and radiation. His mother had diabetes, and he had a couple of negative experiences with doctors while helping her get treatment.

Over time, as he gathered more data to confirm his misgivings, he grew ever more skeptical. Feeling compelled to make up for what medical resources lacked, Tony would give himself screenings on a regular basis, search symptoms on the internet and go to the ER, urgent care or his PCP for any new bodily sensation. Dissatisfied when doctors couldn't give him answers, he often requested a variety of tests, depending on the symptom, and switched doctors frequently. Seeing how much Tony's underlying belief was making his life harder, we decided to do a cost–benefit analysis of its impact on his life. See the results in Table 1. Also, please review the steps for this exercise on page 133 of Chapter 6.

The maladaptive belief: *Medical providers, tests and treatments are wholly incompetent, ineffective and will be unable to help me detect or treat a disease.*

Advantages of maladaptive belief:

- It motivates me to stay on top of my health because believing that those in the healthcare setting can't help me makes me feel compelled to take care of everything myself. *REFRAME: I am not sure if I am 'staying on top of my health' just because I check my body multiple times a day, go to the doctor for every little thing, get lots of tests and google symptoms all the time. So far, all of my excessive behavior hasn't helped me be healthier. It has mostly just made me miserable.*
- By not accepting a doctor's assessment and challenging them, it keeps them on their toes and might keep them from making mistakes or being lazy or not thinking of the right test or the underlying disease that may be causing the symptom. *REFRAME: Although there can be value in being thorough in communicating concerns or bringing additional information to the doctor, a lot of times this doesn't give me the answers I am hoping for or add value in the way I think it will. I run out of time or the test or my suggestions from the internet aren't necessarily helpful. We both end up frustrated and I still don't feel relief because sometimes certain symptoms can't be explained. A more balanced approach might be more helpful (both accepting their assessment and giving my feedback about concerns).*
- When I get multiple scans or other tests just to be safe (because I worry the test results are wrong), I am being preventative. *REFRAME: Even though there are cases in which extra testing is warranted, I haven't yet been given reason to think this is true for me. It would be better to only do extra scans when necessary, such as when it is indicated by family history, DNA testing or a concerning symptom, instead of 'just because.'*

Disadvantages of holding the maladaptive belief:

- I am tired of feeling angry, anxious, out of control, frustrated and just plain exhausted all the time. It's hard to accept a doctor's assessment or a test result, so I feel no relief. I am always unsatisfied and wondering about whether the physician asked the right questions, ordered the right test or whether the test itself is reliable.
- My interactions with medical providers are not always positive (my skepticism is sometimes obvious, I ask a lot of questions and they run out of time and have to cut me off and then I feel more disappointed, dissatisfied and frustrated). It strains my relationship with them and makes me not want to go back. This makes me want to switch doctors often, which makes everything harder—I have to get records transferred, start over and explain everything again.
- I've started dreading doctor appointments because all the negative emotions take up so much of my energy, so I find that if I have an appointment in the middle of the day, I spend the whole morning in dread of going to that appointment.
- Because I doubt that the medical field would be able to help me if I did get diagnosed with a major disease, it makes diseases seem that much scarier. I assume they won't catch it in time or the treatment won't work so any disease will kill me.
- My doubt and lack of trust lead me to take matters into my own hands a lot by checking my body or googling everything, which only makes me more anxious. In other words, these beliefs make me act in ways that I know aren't good for my mental health.
- I have read that it is not good to expose your body to too many scans and I have had a lot of them.
- My skepticism costs me a lot of money. I often go to multiple doctors to get the answers I am looking for because I assume a doctor isn't being thorough enough. I also request a lot of tests and some of them aren't covered by insurance. I have spent thousands of dollars over time on extra tests and doctor visits, urgent care or ER visits.
- Lately, my kids are always asking me if I am okay. They hear me talk about doctors and medical tests with my wife a LOT. I think it is starting to make them feel more anxious and worry that something is really wrong with me.

- I consult a lot with family and friends about my concerns and whether they think the doctors are right or the tests are valid. I can tell they are getting tired of it and it is impacting our relationship. I'm also becoming the 'boy who cried wolf' so to speak.

Holding a revised, more adaptive belief: *Many medical providers, tests and treatments are effective and capable of helping me detect and treat a disease. I can put a reasonable amount of trust in the field to help me, while still advocating for myself and making accommodations as necessary.*

Advantages of holding the more adaptive belief:

- I would feel happier in general because I wouldn't be consumed by anger, doubt, frustration, anxiety and stress. I think I would feel 'lighter.'
- I wouldn't dread doctor appointments anymore and so I would be able to enjoy the hours leading up to the appointment and live like a normal person (e.g. enjoy work and lunch before my 1pm doc appointment). Days that I have medical appointments could actually feel like normal days.
- If I was able to trust or relax a little more, I wouldn't feel the need to do so many extra things for my health. This would allow me to spend more time doing things that make me happy and fulfilled, like spending time with my family, golfing, fantasy football and working out.
- If I didn't feel the need to spend so much money on medical visits and tests, I would be able to pay off some of our credit card debt. This would alleviate financial stress and would help me feel a little freer.
- I could actually feel relieved after getting the results of a physical, screening or test. I haven't had that in a long time. It would be nice to remember what that feels like.
- Doctor appointments wouldn't be stressful and take everything out of me.
- If I believed that, at least to a certain extent, medical interventions could identify and manage it if I were to become ill, then I would be less scared of getting sick.

- It would be refreshing to just be able to relax. I could leave some of the decisions to the medical experts and feel comfortable enough to accept their recommendation and roll with it.

Disadvantages of holding the more adaptive belief:

- It is scary to 'trust' doctors or other medical providers and tests when they could fail me. I have heard stories about people getting misdiagnosed or being told a symptom is nothing when it is something serious. I worry that if I just assume that medicine is overall capable and can help me, then I will be let down and my health will suffer as a result. *REFRAME: It can definitely feel frightening to take the first step toward trusting medical providers and tests when it comes to my health but it doesn't have to be blind trust. I can trust while also giving input and even seeking a second opinion as necessary. I can start with small, baby steps. If it turns out I am let down, I can take the necessary next steps to address the problem.*
- What if I ease up about all of this and then become just a passive person who gets lost in the healthcare system and misses the signs of a serious disease? *REFRAME: I need to remember that I am in control. Just because I decided to trust a little more does not mean I will go to the other extreme and do nothing about symptoms. I can think of this change as not black and white but more about changing where I am on a spectrum. I will move closer to the middle of the spectrum but it doesn't mean I am all the way over on the other extreme. I know how to advocate for myself and will continue to do so if necessary. The idea is to take reasonable steps instead of excessive steps. But I can ease up in small ways as a place to start.*
- I will have a hard time living with so much more uncertainty. I already have a hard time with any uncertainty. Accepting results of doctor assessments and tests means being even less certain and I don't know if I can handle that. *REFRAME: It will definitely take effort to become more comfortable with uncertainty around this. But in reality I can't achieve certainty anyway, even with all the things I do when I don't feel doubtful or skeptical. So either way, I have to live with some uncertainty. Also, I can continue to work on my skills around accepting uncertainty which will make it easier over time. I can build my 'uncertainty muscle' slowly and steadily, over time.*

Tony's results

This exercise allowed Tony to see the profound negative impact his belief was having on his life. All of the problematic thoughts, unpleasant feelings and unhelpful behaviors were in direct response to his assumption that the field of medicine wouldn't be able to help him identify or cope with a disease.

Tony's analysis of his belief (i.e. *medicine is ineffective and will be unable to help him*) revealed that the disadvantages (60) outweighed the advantages (40). In addition, after reviewing the costs and benefits of holding a revised, more adaptive belief (i.e. *having a reasonable amount of trust that the field would be able to help him detect and treat a disease*), he determined that the benefits or advantages (70) of holding this belief outweighed the costs (30). This exercise allowed Tony to see a detailed illustration of how his sweeping generalizations about medicine were harming him more than they were protecting him. This exercise motivated Tony to work on revising his beliefs so that he could improve his quality of life.

Exploring your beliefs about medicine

Not surprisingly, those who have faced trauma or adversity in the medical setting are particularly vulnerable to the development of problematic core beliefs. Any type of trauma can break one's sense of safety, trust, personal agency and value.[7] Medical trauma can be particularly complicated in that one must continue to engage with and rely on the very system that the traumatic event occurred in.[4] In addition, more generally, given the flawed state of whatever healthcare system you are a part of, we all, to varying degrees, will face challenges when it comes to accessing healthcare. Still, despite the flaws and consequential challenges, it is necessary to develop more helpful views of medicine, if only for the mere purpose of not allowing your beliefs to interfere with getting the care you need.

See Table 1 below for some examples of unhelpful beliefs about medicine that can lead to problematic thoughts and behaviors. As you read through the list in Table 1, try to think of any additional problematic beliefs you may have that aren't listed here.

Table 1 Examples of unhelpful or maladaptive beliefs about medicine

- Doctors/medical providers are rude, inconsiderate and lack compassion.
- Doctors/medical professionals always have an agenda and don't care about my wishes.
- Doctors/medical providers are untrustworthy and only in it for the money.
- Doctors/medical providers are lazy, careless and cut corners.
- Doctors/medical providers are incompetent and ineffective.
- If a doctor/medical provider refers me for a medical test, then something must be seriously wrong with me.
- Doctors/medical providers should be able to identify/explain the origin of all bodily sensations/symptoms.
- Medical tests are invalid and unreliable and are likely to miss something.
- Medical interventions/treatments are ineffective and will likely not help me.
- Medical interventions/treatments harm more than help people.

Note that a key difference between adaptive and maladaptive beliefs is the *rigidity* in the language. We want to stay away from overgeneralizations or black-and-white thinking. For example, perhaps a medical provider made egregious mistakes while treating you. Such an awful experience is valid and that medical provider was, indeed, ineffective. However, we need to refrain from overgeneralizing and assuming that *all* or *most* doctors are similarly ineffective. This overgeneralization is what we want to target because it can lead to all sorts of problems in life.

Table 2 illustrates examples of some more adaptive beliefs. Keep in mind that these two tables are not exhaustive lists of adaptive and maladaptive beliefs.

Table 2 Examples of more helpful or adaptive beliefs about medicine

- Although not all, many doctors/medical providers are competent, capable and make sound, evidence-informed decisions.
- Although not all, many doctors/medical providers are patient-centered, compassionate and aim to respect my treatment preferences whenever possible.
- A doctor may order a test simply to follow policy/standard protocols or best practices, not necessarily because they are convinced something is wrong.
- Medical tests are often based on extensive research and best practice recommendations. Tests, scans, examinations are used because they have been shown to be valid and reliable. In the majority of cases, medical tests are accurate.
- Due to the advancement of medicine, there are viable treatment options and resources to help me overcome and/or cope with the majority of illnesses.

Exploring the impact of medical trauma/adversity

If you have had a traumatic or adverse experience in the medical setting, it can be helpful to explore what happened and how this event/events have impacted you. Take a few minutes to reflect on the questions in Table 3 and write your trauma narrative. You don't need to answer every question but focus on the ones that resonate and help guide you in developing your trauma narrative. *Note, if it is too difficult to review the specifics of the experience right now, you can simply focus on the impact alone and not the details about the event itself.*

Table 3 Writing your trauma/adversity narrative

- What happened? Are you still in the middle of this?
- How was this experience for you (or these experiences)? What were your thoughts and feelings during the event? What was your reaction, both in the moment, directly afterward, and up until now?
- Who was present during and after?
- Do you find yourself thinking about what you or others could have/should have done differently? How do these thoughts impact you?
- Do you find yourself thinking about how this experience could have been prevented? How do these thoughts impact you?
- Do you find yourself thinking about why this happened to you? How have these thoughts impacted you?
- How has your experience impacted how you view yourself, others, the world and the future?
- Has this experience impacted your sense of safety? How so?
- Has this experience impacted your ability to trust (yourself and/or others)? How so?
- Has this experience made you feel powerless and out of control? How so?
- Has this experience impacted your belief in others' capability? How so?
- Has this experience impacted your current daily living or plans for the future? How so?
- Has this experience impacted your relationships/connections with others? How so?
- How has this experience impacted your sense of independence and belief in your capability and self-sufficiency?
- How has this experience impacted your view of yourself and relationship with yourself?
- Has this experience impacted your career, relationships with loved ones, ability to enjoy hobbies and overall life satisfaction? How so?
- Has this experience triggered/brought up any previous trauma or adversity in your life (e.g. digging up old wounds related to powerlessness, trust, etc.)?
- Has this experience changed the way you understand or value life and mortality?

For some people, it can be helpful to read this narrative to a close, trusted loved one, such as a partner, relative or close friend. Of course, it is perfectly okay if you do not feel comfortable with that at this point. Regardless, if you have experienced a medical trauma or adversity, it will be useful to keep this trauma narrative in mind while we work through the various strategies in this chapter (as well as in Chapter 10).

Beliefs about medicine and thinking errors

Let's now discuss what can happen when we do develop unhelpful or maladaptive core beliefs. When we hold rigid beliefs that doctors, tests and treatments will be unable to help us detect or treat a disease, this can result in thinking errors when it comes to our interpretation of situations in our daily lives.

To illustrate, if you hold the belief that *doctors are more likely than not to make mistakes regarding my health*, then you might question everything your doctor tells you about a new symptom or your overall health. If you believe that *medical tests are invalid, unreliable and should not be trusted*, you likely will have a difficult time accepting the results of a test. If you believe, *if I develop or contract a disease, there won't be much that can be done to help me cope with or overcome it*, you will likely be even more afraid when a new symptom pops up because any potential disease will presumably result in a catastrophic outcome. Below are a few examples of my clients' (as well as my) problematic thoughts while interacting with the medical system.

Catastrophizing: Predicting only the most disastrous outcomes when it comes to diagnosis and medical care. One will be misdiagnosed and/or treatment will fail to save them.

Many people with health anxiety fear having an undetected disease. I've often been guilty of catastrophizing about a test missing a serious diagnosis. After I had a breast ultrasound to examine a lump, the radiologist came into the room to talk to me about her assessment. She told me that it was highly unlikely that the lump was cancerous and proceeded to explain all the reasons they believed it was a benign cyst. However, she said just in case, we would have a follow-up ultrasound in two months. The 'just in case' sent me down a rabbit hole. I wondered, what exactly does 'in case' mean here? In case I come back in two months to find that, oopsie daisy, looks like we were wrong after all and it is, indeed, cancer? But, of course, by that point it would have spread everywhere and I'd have just a few months to live. I ended up getting more testing and a second opinion and the new radiologist came to the same conclusion.

Not only was I catastrophizing that the test would fail to identify a cancerous lump, but I also assumed that in two months, the cancer would spread everywhere and I would die. As stated before, misdiagnoses do happen, tests cannot guarantee 100 percent accuracy and second opinions are necessary at times. However, we move into problematic thinking when we assume that these catastrophic outcomes are likely.

> All-or-nothing thinking: Viewing health, diagnosis and medical treatment in only two categories. One either has no medical conditions and is healthy and 'safe' or they have a medical condition and are facing death and 'in danger.'

One reason many of my health-anxious clients fear getting a disease is because they have a hard time trusting the adequacy of medical resources to treat it. My client, Jessie, had a debilitating fear of receiving a cancer diagnosis. When I asked why the threat of getting cancer seemed so insurmountable, she explained to me, matter-of-factly, that a cancer diagnosis meant death and leaving her son behind. She moved instantly from diagnosis to dead-in-a-casket. We explored this and discovered that the few stories she'd heard over the years of people only living weeks past a cancer diagnosis stuck with her.

Over time, she focused more on these situations than the many other situations she knew of in which someone received adequate treatment. She began to assume failed treatment was the norm and would be the most likely outcome if she ever faced cancer. It became difficult for her to accept the more likely situation that many medical interventions would lie on the spectrum between her receiving a cancer diagnosis and death. We worked on helping Jessie revise her view to see that, due to the advancement of medicine, there will likely be viable treatment options and resources available to help her overcome or manage and cope with a variety of diseases.

> Overgeneralization: Making a broad negative conclusion about all medical providers or experiences in the medical setting based on one or a few situations.

Some people have frightening and traumatic experiences in the medical setting. My client, Deon, had an unsettling experience with her gynecologist. In a rude and condescending manner, her pain symptoms were dismissed as being a normal part of menstruation and presumed to be related to stress. She was not referred for any testing. After switching to a new gynecologist, Deon discovered she had a cyst that was causing the pain. After being patronized and dismissed, Deon found it difficult to trust doctors and she began to believe that medical providers, in general, were careless, incompetent and lacked compassion.

Gradually, her health anxiety worsened and she started to avoid medical care. In our therapy sessions, Deon and I worked on helping her revise these assumptions. Despite having had a demoralizing and unacceptable experience with the first doctor she consulted, Deon was able to recognize that other medical providers she has interacted with have been compassionate, thorough and effective.

Jumping to conclusions: Making assumptions about a future event without substantial evidence or when evidence supports the contrary.

Experiencing a traumatic medical event can lead one to attempt to gain back a sense of control in their life by trying to anticipate or know what will happen. My client, Andie, had a traumatic childbirth experience. She and her baby almost died, which resulted in an emergency C-section. Fortunately, Andie and her baby were both okay but due to the medical complications that arose, she had to stay in the hospital for several extra days. Andie's pregnancy was uncomplicated and she planned to have a vaginal birth until this unexpected event took place.

Understandably, Andie was shaken by this sudden experience. She began having panic attacks and severe health anxiety shortly afterward. Andie had also been dealing with a knee injury and had a couple of minor procedures, which were scheduled to take place a couple of months after the birth. She canceled both procedures, convinced that something would unexpectedly go wrong during the procedures, as it did during childbirth. In our work together, I helped Andie learn how to refrain from jumping to conclusions about all medical procedures and slowly begin facing her fears in baby steps.

Identifying triggers and thoughts

An important first step is to identify events or situations related to the medical setting that trigger your health anxiety and the thoughts you have in response to these triggers. This can be particularly helpful if you have experienced a traumatic or adverse event in the medical setting. Identifying triggers and thought patterns can help you identify the thoughts that cause you distress, lead to unhelpful behaviors and/or reactivate any traumatic experiences you have had. Of course, this is not an exhaustive list but just a few examples. Take note of any that resonate and feel free to think of additional ones.

Table 4 Examples of triggers

Sensory reminders	Certain sights (e.g. seeing blood, medical devices or procedures, needles, an ambulance or fire truck, bright or flashing lights, fluorescent lights similar to those in a hospital, hospital rooms or beds, medical scenes in a movie or show); certain noises (e.g. hearing someone's medical story, someone's voice, whispering, sounds of medical devices or procedures such as taping or wrapping a wound, the sound of an urgent situation or emergency, office phones ringing); certain smells (e.g. disinfectant, wounds); the way something feels (e.g. certain textures, being touched in a certain place like where an injury happened); the way something tastes (e.g. food that reminds you of being in the hospital)
Situations	Going into a medical setting for any reason (e.g. medical emergencies, medical appointments, visiting others or work); calling to make medical appointments or discuss test results, receiving a call, text or email from a medical provider; taking medication; interactions with staff from insurance companies; interactions with staff regarding financials or paying medical bills
Internal experiences	Disconcerting thoughts or images; experiencing intense emotions that remind you of a past experience; experiencing bodily sensations that remind you of a past medical event or mean you will have to make an appointment/interact with the medical setting

Hopefully, you have an idea of some of the events or stimuli that trigger your health anxiety. I'd like you to begin the habit of recognizing how these triggers have impacted your thoughts. Knowing how this has played out in the past will help you to recognize these patterns in real time. For example, let's say receiving a call, email or text from your doctor's office reminds you of a past frightening experience. This triggers a sense of overwhelming anxiety, and you spiral anytime you receive a message from a healthcare facility, even if it is just a reminder for your annual screening. Your catastrophic thoughts then lead you to avoid communication with anyone at the healthcare facility.

To improve this unhelpful pattern, you'll want to identify the thought patterns that are connected to any triggers for your health anxiety. Similar to what we have done in other chapters, you'll want to also evaluate your thoughts in response to these triggers and look for any distortions or thinking errors. It can also be helpful to recognize whether and how any of your thoughts link back to core beliefs about medicine. Again, these core beliefs could be related to any adverse or traumatic medical events or they could just be beliefs you hold because you fear having an adverse or traumatic medical event. Regardless, it is necessary to become aware of how your triggers, thought patterns and underlying core beliefs about medicine are all connected. See the list of thinking errors and a thought record with examples below.

Common thinking errors

- All-or-nothing thinking
- Jumping to conclusions
- Catastrophizing
- Emotional reasoning
- Mental filter/Tunnel vision
- Unrealistic expectations
- Overgeneralization
- Magical thinking

Record to identify triggers, thoughts & underlying beliefs

Date, trigger & unpleasant emotion rating (1–10)

March 22

Had to go to the ER due to an injury from a minor car accident.

Anxiety: 8/10
Anger: 9/10

Automatic thought in response to the trigger or situation

I am not going to get the care that I need. They either are going to overlook something or treat me poorly and I am going to feel stressed out on top of not getting my injury adequately addressed.

Level of concern: 9/10

Did this trigger or situation remind me of any past events? Did it trigger a sense of powerlessness, lack of safety, distrust, insecurity?

Being in the ER and hearing all of the chaos/hurried medical staff reminded me of when I came in years ago with abdominal pain, indigestion and nausea. A medical provider was dismissive about my symptoms and questioned why I came into the ER for a stomach ache instead of my PCP. After I pushed back and advocated for myself to get further assessment, I was diagnosed with a stomach ulcer. Entering the ER for an injury reminded me of feeling powerless and not being able to trust the last time I came to the ER. I felt unsafe, like I wasn't going to get the help I needed.

Potential thinking errors

(1) Jumping to conclusions: assuming that a certain outcome will take place—that medical providers will overlook my injury and/or will treat me poorly—when I don't yet have evidence or reason to believe that this will happen.

(2) Tunnel vision: focusing on the one terrible experience I had, while not considering the other neutral or positive experiences I have had while receiving healthcare.

Underlying core beliefs (whether impacted by a past medical trauma or not): Core beliefs that were behind my triggers/thoughts included beliefs that all or most medical providers are unkind, untrustworthy and incompetent. It led me to instantly feel anxious upon entering the ER because I anticipated having to deal with a similar experience.

Date, trigger & unpleasant emotion rating (1–10)

May 14

Got an ultrasound due to abnormal periods. A small cyst was noted but determined to be benign. Doctor recommended to 'follow' the cyst and will get periodic imaging to assess for any changes.

Anxiety: 9/10

Automatic thought in response to the trigger or situation

How can he know for sure that it is benign? What if he is just being lazy and doesn't want to deal with looking further into this? I have a feeling this could be something more. I've heard stories about lazy assessments and misdiagnoses.

Level of concern: 10/10

Did this trigger or situation remind me of any past events? Did it trigger a sense of powerlessness, lack of safety, distrust, insecurity?

I haven't had personal experiences with medical trauma/ adversity, such as having a diagnosed medical condition, being misdiagnosed or having difficult or frightening experiences in the medical setting, but I have heard stories about these things happening to people. I have read articles and heard stories from people I am acquainted with or on social media. Hearing this has made me have trouble trusting a doctor's assessment.

Potential thinking errors

(1) Emotional reasoning: believing the cyst is something more serious simply because it feels true, even when evidence points to the contrary (the dimensions of the cyst are consistent with benign cysts).

(2) Unrealistic expectations: assuming that if a doctor can't tell me with 100 percent certainty (that the cyst is benign), then the doctor/test isn't to be trusted.

(3) Mental filter: only remembering all of the stories of misdiagnoses and failing to acknowledge all of the examples of people who were accurately diagnosed and treated.

Underlying core beliefs (whether impacted by a past medical trauma or not): I struggle with believing that doctors and tests are untrustworthy. These beliefs make it difficult to trust or accept the results of any test or anything a doctor concludes based on their assessment. I find that I have a general pattern of doing this, such as doubting the results when I get my annual physical blood work or routine screenings like a mammogram, colonoscopy, etc.

Using Socratic dialogue to challenge thoughts about medicine

The next step after building awareness of your thought patterns when it comes to doctors, tests and treatments is to challenge any unhelpful or maladaptive thoughts. Again, this isn't to say that we want you to have blind trust in every doctor, test or treatment option. There are times when second opinions are not only necessary but essential, especially if you are investigating a complicated health concern or deciding which treatment option is best for you. That said, we don't want ongoing distorted or unhelpful thinking patterns to reinforce a general pattern of mistrust and doubt. These thought patterns make you more anxious and lead to unhealthy behaviors, such as the *overuse* of medical care (safety behaviors) or *underuse* of medical care (avoidance).

We will now continue the practice of using Socratic dialogue to help you challenge thinking errors and reshape unhelpful thinking patterns. In this chapter we will help you learn to challenge thoughts related to the general pattern of fear, doubt and mistrust when it comes to interacting with the medical setting. If it helps, review the section in Chapter 3 on why and how using this strategy can help you reshape biases and distorted thinking.

Draw from the questions below as inspiration to help you critically analyze your thoughts and seek out any potential inconsistencies, contradictions or exceptions. We simply want you to modify any unhelpful thoughts and assumptions that might be negatively impacting your relationship with healthcare. Remember, not all questions will be relevant to you so focus only on those that are helpful for you and try to come up with additional questions.

Examples of Socratic questions related to the distrust and doubt in the medical setting

- What specifically am I afraid will happen in the medical setting? What is the evidence for this? Is there any evidence against it? In other words, is there any evidence for a different, better outcome?
- How does assuming or living in fear of this experience or outcome impact my life? What could be the benefits of having a little trust or hope that it will turn out okay?

- Are my fears and assumptions based on extreme or black-and-white thinking? Am I using terms like all, every/none, need/have to, always/never, must/must not, can't, should/shouldn't? Is there a more balanced, middle-road way of seeing this?
- How much is the intolerance of uncertainty playing a role in my ability to accept a doctor's assessment or the results of a test? Am I having a difficult time accepting any uncertainty or hoping to be 100 percent guaranteed that a test or assessment is correct? Can I work toward becoming comfortable with the likely probability that a test result is accurate without the need for a guarantee?
- Are my fears and assumptions leading me to jump to conclusions about a situation? For example, am I jumping to conclusions about the inaccuracy of a test or doctor's assessment without adequate evidence? Can I momentarily set my fear aside and look only at the facts? Can I work on accepting results unless or until new information tells me to do otherwise?
- How much are my feelings driving my fear and doubt over having a negative or catastrophic experience while receiving healthcare? For example, if going to the doctor or to a hospital triggers me and causes a lot of anxiety, how much importance am I putting on these feelings? Am I incorrectly assuming feelings are facts and making interpretations about future events based on the way that I am feeling?
- Am I engaging in tunnel vision and basing my fears of being mistreated, dismissed, misdiagnosed or inadequately treated on one or two situations I have heard of or witnessed? Am I giving a fair amount of attention or consideration to all of the other neutral or positive experiences in healthcare? Can I draw from these other situations to help me form a more balanced perspective?
- Am I confusing something that is possible with something that is likely? What is the likelihood of my fear?
- If I were to have a negative experience in the medical setting (medical trauma or adversity), am I assuming the outcome will be catastrophic? In what ways might the situation be negative and difficult but not catastrophic?
- Let's put your feared event on a spectrum. On one side, write out the worst-case scenario. On the other side of the spectrum, write out the best-case scenario. Remember to be intentional about thinking 'big'

when it comes to the best-case scenario (we need to make up for the tendency to spend most of our energy/time near the worst-case scenario). Now, circle the area in the middle of the spectrum and write out the most common scenario. What is the middle-of-the-spectrum, most likely outcome in this situation?

- If I were to have a negative experience in the medical setting (medical trauma or adversity), how could I cope with this difficult experience? What actionable steps could I take to manage this type of situation (e.g. advocate for myself, involve others, get another provider or second opinion, explore various treatment options)? What social, cultural, spiritual, emotional/psychological resources would help me cope with challenging situations?
- If I have had a traumatic or adverse experience in the medical setting, how much does this influence my fears? Am I seeing the future through the lens of my traumatic experience and assuming I will be subjected to it again? Am I overly focused on this one experience (tunnel vision) and drawing broad conclusions from it (overgeneralization)? How can I make space for the possibility of a different experience? Outside of my negative experience(s), have I had neutral or positive experiences in the medical setting (e.g. a medical issue is accurately identified and adequately addressed, my concerns are heard, positive or neutral interactions with healthcare professionals)?
- If I have had a traumatic or adverse experience in the medical setting, how did I cope with this? What helped me to get through it? What did I learn? How can I draw from my strength, resilience and new knowledge to cope with anything that happens in the future?

Modifying biased information processing

When we hold a belief, we selectively attend to information in our environment that supports that belief. Thus, if we believe that the entire medical system will fail to help us detect or treat a disease, we will search for, or at the very least are more likely to notice, data in our environment that reinforces the belief (e.g. someone gets misdiagnosed, a medical intervention failed to save someone). We are also more likely to ignore or dismiss data in our environment that challenges the belief (e.g. a thorough doctor identifies a health concern, someone is living a fulfilling life in the midst of managing a chronic illness).

For example, I have an odd interest in watching videos and reading stories about plane crashes that have happened across the world (yes, I know this little hobby does not help my anxiety and, yes, I am working on it). Periodically, however, I sink back into this old pattern of behavior. When I slipped back into this habit recently, I was in for a treat, given the algorithmic world we now live in. I became inundated with stories about plane crashes and other scary plane incidents on social media and in my newsfeed on my phone. After a couple of weeks of this, these events started to seem inevitable! However, we all know this isn't true. It is generally accepted that flying in a commercial airplane is by far the safest form of travel available. Yet, if you flood your brain with enough of something, you can really start to get a warped view of reality.

But you can make changes to this process by being intentional about the environmental stimuli that you pay attention to as well as how you process that information. Although we know, for example, that our medical system in the United States is far from perfect, at the same time we don't want you assuming it is utterly useless and incapable of helping you manage your health. Thus, instead of thinking in black-and-white terms in either direction (medicine is flawless, medicine is useless), the goal is to help you see medicine in a more balanced, adaptive way. To oversimplify it, if we were to place your view of medicine on the spectrum below, we'd want you to move closer to the middle of the spectrum or beyond.

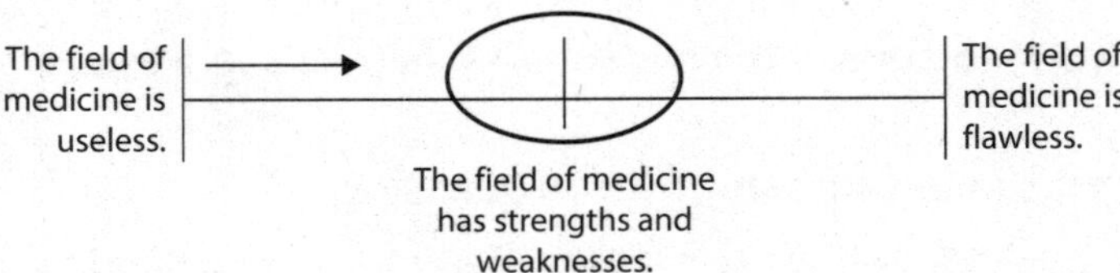

The field of medicine is useless.
The field of medicine is flawless.
The field of medicine has strengths and weaknesses.

To accomplish this goal, I am going to teach you a few strategies in this section to help you be more intentional about how you gather and interpret information in your day-to-day life. Each of these strategies will help you build awareness of your tendencies as well as help you to be more deliberate and gain some control over this process.

Content cleanse

One strategy you can use to improve this tendency is the content cleanse we used in Chapter 3 in which you become intentional about *limiting* the content you consume and what you surround yourself with every day. See Chapter 3 for a refresher on this exercise. As we did before, take inventory of the different ways you consume this type of content on a regular basis.

I will give you a few examples from my client, Casey.

- Reading stories about negative experiences in healthcare on Quora
- Reading articles about people who died from cancer after treatment failed
- Watching videos on TikTok and Instagram about people's tragic personal stories with terminal disease
- Reading comment sections in videos on social media, many people complaining about medical providers being incompetent and uncaring
- Watching news clips or YouTube videos about negative experiences in healthcare
- Seeking out conversations with people at church or at work about negative experiences in the medical setting

Once you have your list, develop your plan for how you will implement the content cleanse. Then select an accountability partner. Remember, this exercise is to help develop a more balanced view of medicine by not spending all of your time on one side of the argument. We will illustrate with Casey's example.

Table 5 My content-consumption limitation plan

Accountability partner: My best friend				
Consumption behavior	Current frequency of this behavior	How this consumption behavior impacts me	Limitation plan	Ways that I will limit behavior or helpful steps I can take
Watching videos on Instagram and TikTok about people who have been misdiagnosed.	Lately, videos pop up on my feed (almost daily) and I usually watch the entire video (or most of the video) when they do pop up.	I've started to become convinced that misdiagnoses are inevitable, which has made me more anxious about my health because I assume I am the only one who will be able to detect a disease. So I have become even more hypervigilant about every symptom lately.	I will try to scroll past these videos whenever they pop up. I will also put other safeguards in place to prevent being inundated with videos like these.	*Safeguards:* 1. I will click 'not interested' in the lower right-hand corner of the video and then click 'topic doesn't interest me' as the reason. 2. I will click 'block' or 'mute' the person (or hide the video) so that this and other similar videos don't show up in my feed.

Table 6 Record of experiences in limiting content consumption

Consumption behavior plan	Log of experiences in limiting the behavior
Limiting watching videos on TikTok/Instagram	It was really hard to do at first. I failed to follow through a couple of times because a couple of really interesting videos popped up and it was hard for me not to watch. But in the past few days I have been really good. I've noticed that after about a week of not watching videos (or clicking 'not interested'), fewer videos are popping up, which is nice because it makes it less tempting. Also, I've been checking in with my best friend every night about whether I watched videos that day and that has helped me.

The 'interview' experiment

With the content cleanse, we modified information processing by being mindful of, and subsequently limiting, information that reinforces unhelpful beliefs. With the interview experiment, we will tackle this issue from a different angle and intentionally seek out data for the other side of the argument—that *there is reason to build some trust in the capacity of medicine to help detect and overcome or manage the vast majority of illnesses.*

Recall that we did a similar interview experiment in Chapter 4. In this case, we want to learn from people who can share neutral or positive experiences in the medical setting, whether through interactions with medical providers or while navigating testing, assessment and/or treatment. For those of us with a 'mixed bag' of experiences while receiving healthcare, it can also be helpful to learn about experiences that were negative at times but turned out okay. The goal, really, is simply to be intentional about paying attention to a different narrative from what normally grasps your attention.

Think of a few people you could interview about their experiences in the medical setting. These experiences could be routine experiences in healthcare (e.g. routine screenings and physicals, seeking consultation or treatment for mild/minor health issues) or they could be more in-depth experiences, such as getting assessment and intervention for medical crises and/or acute or chronic medical conditions. You will want to learn about the help they received during these (potentially difficult) experiences. In other words, you'll want to know about how the setting, medical providers and interventions gave them any amount of encouragement, relief and/or hope.

Select three to five people who are willing to share their experiences. Remember, the goal of this exercise is to hear the other side of the story, about neutral or positive experiences in healthcare. Thus, you want to be selective for this interview. If you know someone who has shared a lot about their awful experiences, opt for someone else with a fresh perspective. Most of us don't have all positive or all negative experiences, so anyone you interview will likely have a range of different experiences. For now, keep your focus on neutral or positive experiences. Below are a few suggestions for interview questions. Of course, feel free to include any additional questions that might help you build a little more trust in the ability of medicine to help you detect or treat illnesses.

Table 7 Sample interview invitation and questions

Sample invitation script: I am interested in learning more about experiences within the medical setting. Now, recognizing that many of us may have had negative experiences of one kind or another over our lifetime, in this exercise I am interested in learning more about either neutral or positive experiences while interacting with the healthcare system. I will, therefore, be asking questions about your interactions with medical providers or through screening, assessment or diagnosis or treatment. Would you be interested in participating in this type of interview?
Example of prompts/topics for interview:
• An experience in which a medical provider went above and beyond the call of duty in some way. • An experience in which a medical provider showed compassion or made you feel heard, validated and/or respected. • An experience in which a medical provider was thorough and/or thoughtful during a screening or physical or in their assessment of a health concern. • An experience in which a medical provider demonstrated competency and knowledge. • An experience in which a medical provider took the time to explain something to you during a medical visit, while getting testing or treatment, or during diagnosis/treatment. • An experience in which a medical provider/assessment/test identified something that you hadn't thought of or that was previously missed. • An experience in which a medical provider advocated for/supported you. • An experience in which an assessment/test accurately identified a medical issue. • An experience in which tests/scans were able to accurately rule out a health concern. • An experience in which an intervention/treatment was effective at helping you to overcome or manage a disease and/or symptoms. • An experience in which medical care helped you to improve your quality of life.

A few reflection questions to consider after the interviews

1. What were some of the key takeaway messages about their experiences in the medical setting?
2. Did you learn anything that surprised you? Did you learn anything that inspired you or helped put things into perspective?
3. Was there anything that resonated with you in particular (e.g., an experience that stood out to you or a specific outlook someone shared that you think might be helpful for you)?
4. How can you integrate what you learned about peoples' experiences in the medical setting into your views about the medical setting or predictions about future experiences?

5 Did anything you learn make you reconsider any unhelpful views about medicine (e.g. that maybe not all doctors/tests/treatments are invalid/useless)?
6 Considering what you learned in this interviews, what might be a more balanced or nuanced view of the field of medicine?

The core belief exercise

My client, Veronica, assumed that she was especially weak and vulnerable to illness, despite any real evidence, and doubted the capability of doctors and medical interventions to 'save' her if she were to be diagnosed with something serious. Of course, as you probably know by now, these beliefs led Veronica to live in fear of her symptoms since she remained convinced that any diagnosis would mean 'the end.'

Veronica and I completed a core belief exercise to explore her reasoning and put any biased thoughts to the test. To refresh your memory on the specific steps (and tips) for successfully completing the core belief exercise, refer back to page 65 in Chapter 3. This exercise helped Veronica to not only pay attention to one side of the argument. Although in her experience doctors had made mistakes, after taking the time to identify evidence for an alternative belief, she was able to develop a more nuanced view.

Old core belief

DOCTORS ARE MORE LIKELY THAN NOT TO MAKE MISTAKES REGARDING MY HEALTH

How much do you believe this core belief (*before the intervention*)? (0–100) **80**

EVIDENCE THAT SEEMS TO SUPPORT THE OLD CORE BELIEF (WITH REFRAME)

- I went to the doctor because I was super sick and they told me it was a cold and it turned out to be strep, a double ear infection and bronchitis. *REFRAME: More than likely I went in super early and may not have been able to identify the problem yet. Also, even if a doctor missed something or wasn't thorough enough, that doesn't mean most or all doctors would do the same.*

- My PCP told me I had a terrible disease that could cause uterine tissue to grow in my intestines, but my gynecologist said it really isn't anything serious at all. *REFRAME: PCPs aren't trained in specialty areas and that's why she referred me to a specialist for further guidance. Also, doctors make mistakes and one doctor's mistake doesn't represent all doctors or the entire field.*
- I dislocated my wrist as a kid and the ER doctor told me it was just a fracture. When I went to the orthopedist, he told me it was dislocated, not fractured. *REFRAME: The ER doc is not an orthopedist; that's why I went to a specialist. Although this was a frustrating situation, when I think back, the majority of doctors my loved ones and I have seen have been competent and correct in their assessments/diagnoses.*
- How much do you believe this core belief (*after the intervention*)? (0–100) **30**

New core belief

MOST OF THE TIME, DOCTORS ARE COMPETENT AND MAKE SOUND, EVIDENCE-INFORMED DECISIONS

How much do you believe this core belief (*before the intervention*)? (0–100) **10**

- Every time a doctor has given me a misdiagnosis, it's been a PCP with minimal expertise in that specific area. I have never been misdiagnosed by a specialist.
- Every time I have had an ailment and followed doctor's orders, I have recovered fully.
- I've had lots of medical needs in my life, have followed doctors' advice and I'm still alive!
- I'm not ever stuck just seeing one doctor; if I feel like I'm misdiagnosed, I can see another doctor, particularly a specialist.
- Doctors often consult one another for more difficult problems. Even though I haven't had a major problem, if I did, I'm sure there would be collaboration on a diagnosis if needed. They also make decisions based on a set of standards in their given field/specialty area.
- There are so many medical tools/treatments, most of which I don't even know about, but doctors do know about them (e.g. my dad

required a lot of interventions for his heart that I never would have known existed).

- My dad has a lot of health problems, which have required the use of numerous medical interventions to address a variety of issues over the years. It is pretty amazing how long he has lived, given that he doesn't take great care of his body despite his health issues. A lot of this has been due to the help of many different doctors and all of the assessment, testing and interventions that have been done. He has lived a relatively long life because of the expertise of these different doctors.
- How much do you believe this core belief (*after the intervention*)? (0–100) **60**

Practical steps to have a more functional relationship with healthcare

Many people with health anxiety have strained relationships with their healthcare providers and/or experience difficulty while interacting with the healthcare system. For health-anxious people with *care-seeking* tendencies, the need for repeated reassurance and difficulty accepting uncertainty can deteriorate relationships with providers and make interactions challenging and unproductive. For health-anxious people with *care-avoidant* tendencies, not seeking care for routine screenings or to manage medical conditions can have a detrimental impact on health, lead to more avoidance and distrust, and further alienate one from the healthcare system. What's more, experiencing trauma or adversity in the medical setting can further exacerbate all of these issues and may make it especially difficult to trust providers and the healthcare system as a whole.

Unfortunately, all of this only makes health anxiety worse over time. The more distrust and fear we experience while interacting with the medical setting, the more our fear of disease will grow. Given that we will all inevitably need to access healthcare at some point in our lives to take care of our bodies, it is imperative that we are able to develop a functional relationship with it. This involves building enough trust in the healthcare system to access the care we need and in a way that is as productive as possible.

When relationships with doctors get messy

Healthy or adaptive relationships are those with open communication, mutual respect, reliability and trust, generally speaking. Relationships with doctors or other healthcare providers should reflect these qualities to some degree. Of course, problems that stem from a flawed healthcare system and/or negative or traumatic experiences in the medical setting can make it even more challenging to achieve this type of relationship. Recognizing that all of our situations are different (e.g. our access to healthcare services, our unique medical status and background) and that no relationship is perfect, we want to help you get as close as possible to an adaptive or functional relationship with your providers.

A lot of my clients with *care-seeking* tendencies often return for appointments to seek reassurance about symptoms, including symptoms they have already consulted about before. They might come to appointments with a detailed list of concerns, which is often difficult to accommodate in one visit, given the time constraints imposed by insurance companies. Many also tend to come to appointments already convinced of the diagnosis based on internet searches or other stories they have heard and, thus, struggle to accept a different opinion, ultimately leading to tension and/or conflict with the provider. They also might feel frustrated when doctors can't give them a guarantee that they don't have the feared disease. All of this has led some of my clients to switch providers regularly or 'shop' for a doctor they hope will be able to meet their needs.

Some of these negative interactions may be due to your doctor's mistakes, oversights or poor bedside manner. Although all doctors are required to undergo extensive education and training, they are also human, and even the best can make mistakes. Nonetheless, as with any profession, there are great and not-so-great doctors. In addition, sometimes providers' efforts are hindered by factors related to a flawed healthcare system, such as insurance company constraints. All that said, when I describe the struggles my clients have in their relationships with providers, I am referring to more than one or two isolated incidents. I am talking about a *general pattern* of interactions with providers that are fraught with problems related to trust, communication, collaboration and treatment planning or implementation. It is important to be honest with yourself about whether your interactions suggest this type of pattern.

When my clients exhibit these types of patterns, we work toward making changes in their thoughts, beliefs and behavior to help improve their relationships with providers. Not all of these strategies were necessary for everyone and some of these tips were more helpful for some than others. Given that your health anxiety 'profile' or struggles are unique, focus only on those that are helpful for you. Importantly, these changes do not take place overnight and are accomplished through small (yet intentional and consistent) steps:

- limiting the focus of appointments with providers by prioritizing the main problem to ensure that the issue is able to be addressed in the time allotted
- refraining from repeatedly seeking reassurance for every bodily sensation, particularly sensations or symptoms that have already been addressed (for *care-seeking* types) or learning to face their fears and attend necessary appointments (for those who tend to be *care-avoidant*)
- refraining from becoming too attached to a diagnosis or other information they found on the internet and, instead, bringing concerns and relevant information while being receptive to their doctor's assessment and professional opinion
- accepting a little uncertainty
- communicating effectively during medical appointments (e.g. planning ahead or making a list to get the most out of appointments, taking notes during appointments, being both assertive about voicing questions and concerns as well as receptive and open to provider input during dialogue)
- giving providers a chance to show they are trustworthy before automatically moving on to another provider (note this does not require them to be perfect but worthy of being given some degree of trust in their assessment, judgment, recommendations)
- refraining from relying on urgent care and emergency room visits for reassurance (except in the case of real emergencies or urgent concerns) and to continue building your relationship with your doctor and/or other medical providers through regularly scheduled visits.

Strategies to improve relationships with doctors

It can be helpful to establish and maintain a consistent, ongoing relationship with your primary care doctor, if your insurance coverage and finances permit this. Schedule routine visits with your doctor for physicals, screenings and immunizations. Allow yourself to slowly build trust with one doctor or clinic instead of engaging in doctor shopping or frequently switching doctors. Lastly, refrain from relying on urgent care and the emergency room for symptom concerns and, instead, consult with your primary doctor (when the symptom warrants a doctor visit).

All of this gives your primary care doctor and their team the opportunity to get to know you and your healthcare needs better. It can also help you build a little more trust in your provider over time, which will ultimately improve your health anxiety.

Replacing ER visits with primary care visits when appropriate

Many of my care-seeking clients have trouble discerning what constitutes a medical emergency. They often ask, *how do I know whether a symptom is a true medical emergency or not?* And this is a fair question. After all, if a symptom seems like a crisis, then it makes sense that *not* going to urgent care or the emergency room can seem scary and dangerous.

The problem is that people with health anxiety can often be convinced that they are having a medical crisis when they are not. Excessive and unnecessary emergency room (and urgent care) visits are time-consuming, costly and, ultimately, only increase health anxiety.[8,9] What's more, using the ER as a substitute for your primary care doctor also prevents you from establishing ongoing, routine care with one consistent provider. This will allow your provider to have a more complete picture of you as the 'whole patient' and offer the opportunity to provide more holistic treatment, which is increasingly recognized as a vital strategy to restore health, promote resilience and prevent disease.[10]

For all of these reasons it can be helpful to learn more about how to distinguish between symptoms that are a crisis and those that can be assessed at a doctor's office or even monitored at home. See Table 8 for a list of symptoms that warrant immediate medical attention, according to the American College of Emergency Physicians.[11]

Note that a couple of the symptoms (dizziness, shortness of breath) are also symptoms you can experience as part of the fight-or-flight response. If you tend to have these symptoms in response to being anxious, particularly if these symptoms or concerns have been cleared by your doctor already, these are not a medical emergency for you. Remember, at times your anxiety may tell you that you are in the middle of a medical crisis.

Table 8 Symptoms that call for immediate medical attention

Bleeding that will not stop	Severe or persistent vomiting
Breathing problems (difficulty breathing, shortness of breath)	Sudden injury due to a motor vehicle accident, burns or smoke inhalation, near drowning, a deep or large wound, or other injuries
Change in mental status (such as unusual behavior, confusion, difficulty arousing)	Sudden, severe pain anywhere in the body
Chest pain or discomfort lasting for two minutes or more	Sudden dizziness, weakness, or change in vision
Choking	Swallowing a poisonous substance
Coughing up or vomiting blood	Severe abdominal pain or pressure
Weak or ineffective coughing	Unusual headache
Fainting or loss of consciousness	Inability to speak
Feeling of committing suicide or murder	Swelling of the face, eyes, or tongue
Head or spine injury	Bluish skin color (cyanosis)

If you have specific fears, such as a heart attack or stroke, you are likely to pay selective attention to any related symptoms. If you begin to feel anxious, your anxiety may trigger symptoms that may make you think you will suffocate or have a heart attack. However, if you've seen a doctor for this and there are no concerns, it is important to work on trusting that.

In the case of a true medical emergency, it will likely be very obvious to you and everyone else. It can also be helpful to consider whether other people you know without anxiety would see this symptom as an emergency and go to the ER. Take into consideration all of this information, including the information in Table 8, when you are worried about a symptom.

It is important to have conversations about all of this with your doctor. Discuss the difference between real medical emergencies and symptoms that can either be assessed at an office visit or that can be simply monitored at home. Your doctor will also be able to add any nuances that may be relevant, given your specific medical background. You will see a prompt for having this discussion with your doctor in the worksheet below.

Establishing consistency with your doctor

Scheduling regular appointments with your primary care doctor, rather than relying on emergency medicine, can help you access more consistent, holistic and individualized care as well as give you the opportunity to build some trust with one healthcare team. Of course, the specific frequency, duration and nature of these appointments will look different for everyone, depending on many factors, such as your age, medical background, behavioral tendencies, the healthcare system you are a part of, insurance coverage and your financial situation.

Set an appointment with your primary care provider to start this process. You can set an appointment to specifically discuss the topics in the worksheet below. This can help establish clear expectations about when it is necessary for you to go to the doctor for routine appointments (e.g. physicals, screenings, vaccinations), manage any ongoing medical conditions and consult about new health concerns. If you have care-seeking tendencies, this can help you refrain from frequently seeking reassurance about symptoms from your doctor. If you have care-avoidant tendencies, this can help you follow through with seeing your doctor for the reasons specified.

It can also be empowering to have frank discussions with your doctor about when a health concern is urgent, with regard to your specific circumstances (age, current medical conditions, medical history). These discussions can reduce anxiety over new symptoms and lessen the burden of trying to figure out the best course of action all on your own. Further, it can be beneficial to schedule regular follow-up appointments to check in about health anxiety (that are phased out over time) in the effort to reduce reassurance-seeking between appointments.[12] As a whole, engaging in this process can help you build trust with your doctor. Review the worksheet below and use it as a guide for discussion at your visit.

Improving communication and establishing a plan with my doctor (regarding visits & health concerns)
I will visit my primary care doctor/specialist when I need check-ups and screenings, which may include the following (list frequency for each): • Regular physicals ____________________ • Vaccinations ____________________ • Prescription renewals ____________________

- Regular medical screenings based on age and medical background (e.g. mammogram, colonoscopy, pap smear, prostate exam)

___

- Regular check-ups to monitor ongoing medical condition(s)

___

I will visit my primary care doctor/specialist when I need to inquire about a new symptom that is clearly abnormal/concerning and does not seem to be related to anxiety and stress (e.g. blood in my stool, severe abdominal pain, lump in my breast). Discuss and write out any examples given by the doctor.

___

I will visit my primary care doctor/specialist when I experience symptoms related to a diagnosed medical condition (list/discuss any current medical condition(s), if relevant, and the changes/symptoms that would warrant a new medical visit):

___

Regarding urgent/emergency health concerns that require immediate attention, I will discuss Table 8 with the doctor. I will also discuss any additional examples they may have of medical emergencies, in consideration of my specific health status and medical background.

___

Below is a list of the symptoms I am *currently concerned about or have often been concerned about* in the past. Discuss with my doctor when it is sufficient to simply monitor these symptoms at home (with the use of coping mechanisms such as rest, fluids, over-the-counter medication) versus when it is necessary to come in for a visit (e.g. they worsen or persist beyond a certain period of time, additional symptoms emerge).

___

____

____

I will discuss with my doctor whether it is necessary/helpful to schedule a routine check-in visit (e.g. quarterly) to check in about progress with health anxiety and further discuss/update any of the details in this form. In doing so, the goal would be to limit additional unnecessary visits to the doctor/emergency room for mild symptoms or symptoms that have already been assessed and cleared. *Note, strategies taught in previous chapters might help to accomplish this, such as cognitive strategies for challenging thoughts and learning to wait before seeking reassurance from doctors.*

____

____

____

____

____

Addressing the tendency to avoid healthcare with exposure

Many people with health anxiety avoid the medical setting as an unhelpful coping mechanism. People who have experienced medical trauma or adversity, in particular, find themselves falling into a pattern of avoidance in response to these experiences.[13] They avoid medical care to protect themselves from a feared outcome, such as being told something is wrong with them, having their concerns dismissed or misdiagnosed, being treated poorly or experiencing pain or discomfort. Regardless, this dysfunctional behavior can have dire consequences for their health.

In Chapter 6, we created an exposure hierarchy to reduce the use of safety behaviors and avoidance (to address *care-seeking* and *care-avoidant* tendencies). This will be an extension of that, in which we will create an exposure or fear hierarchy to help you learn how to not avoid getting healthcare. Revisit Chapter 6 (Page 147) to review the steps for designing and implementing your hierarchy.

We discussed Casey earlier in this chapter, whose pain was misdiagnosed by her first doctor. As a result, Casey avoided and delayed medical care. This habit worsened over time. For example, she started avoiding going to the doctor for simple appointments, such as for her annual physical. Or when she noticed a little pain in her shoulder after it had healed, she continued to put off scheduling an appointment even though it would have been prudent for her to check on her shoulder after experiencing pain again.

Casey and I created a fear hierarchy to help her begin to engage with the healthcare system again as necessary. As a first step, we identified her feared consequences, triggers/cues and avoidant behaviors. See Chapter 6 to review tips for completing the table below.

Table 9 Casey's summary of feared consequences, triggers and avoidant behaviors

Feared consequences
• Having her health concerns dismissed/misunderstood and feeling unheard/ invisible, experiencing anger, anxiety and a sense of helplessness and hopelessness • Having a health issue that isn't addressed and causes more suffering • Having a disease that isn't identified and worsens as a result • Being told the scary news that she has a serious health concern.
Cues or triggers related to medical setting
(i.e. what triggers the imagined/feared consequences) • Going into a medical setting for any reason • Waiting rooms in a medical setting • Seeing certain types of expressions on medical providers' faces that seem to indicate confusion, uncertainty or lack of interest, compassion or understanding • Getting scans, bloodwork or other testing done • Awaiting the results of a test (waiting for an email or phone call or doctors walking into the room to give a test result) • Intrusive images or catastrophic thoughts about doctors telling her they don't know what is wrong and will run more tests • Intrusive images or catastrophic thoughts about doctors telling her something is seriously wrong with her • Experiencing any new symptom (but especially shoulder pain) and realizing or fearing having to interact with doctors/medical setting again.
Avoidant behaviors related to medical setting
• Avoid getting physicals or recommended screenings (or put off as long as possible) • Avoid scheduling an appointment when have a new symptom (or put off as long as possible) • Ignore email messages, texts or phone calls from medical offices (for upcoming screenings, follow-up appointments or even related to records/ finance department) • If notice a new symptom or old symptom (such as shoulder pain) that might require me to go to the doctor, avoid thinking about it and try to pretend it isn't there.

It's your turn! Similar to Casey's example, make a table that includes a list for each of these three categories. You will then draw from your table and use it as inspiration for creating an exposure hierarchy.

Table 10 My summary of feared consequences, triggers and avoidant behaviors

My feared consequences
My cues or triggers related to the medical setting
My avoidant behaviors related to the medical setting

Once you have brainstormed and developed your lists, create the exposure or fear hierarchy. Include around 10–20 items that we will place in order, starting with the easiest task (40/100 SUDS) and working our way up to the hardest task (100/100 SUDS). Remember, the items in the list and the order in which they are ranked are unique to everyone, based on specific fears, triggers and behaviors. No two hierarchies will look the same.

Start at the bottom of the hierarchy and work your way up to the top of the hierarchy. Think of this as taking baby steps that will get more challenging as you progress and increase your confidence. Exposure items could be situational, imaginal or interoceptive, depending on your specific fears, triggers and behaviors. The goal is to learn to engage with the healthcare system as necessary even in the face of situations, thoughts or images that remind you of negative experiences and/or trigger your health anxiety. See Casey's hierarchy for an example.

Table 11 Casey's exposure/fear hierarchy

Task #	Casey's fear hierarchy	SUDS
14	Attend my appointment with orthopedist for my shoulder and get information on doctor's assessment and recommendations for continued care.	100/100
13	Answer the phone call/read email/return to doctor to retrieve results for my annual physical/blood work (depending on office policy).	95/100
12	A couple of days before the appointment with the orthopedist for my shoulder pain, I will drive to the office and sit in the waiting room for 20 minutes (I will not be seeing the doctor this time).	85/100
11	Write out an imaginal exposure scenario: Imagine myself going to the orthopedist and explaining the recent symptom of pain. Imagine that I have to clarify my concerns at one point to make sure the doctor understands. Imagine the doctor listens to my concerns and then makes a few recommendations for follow-up assessment or testing. I will read this twice per day until my appointment.	80/100
10	Write out an imaginal exposure scenario: Right after or shortly after I attend my appointment for my annual physical and check-up (i.e. before I get the actual results of the physical), imagine getting the phone call with the test results (or email or going to a follow-up visit depending on the office policy for obtaining results). Imagine answering the call or opening the email and getting test results that indicate a few minor concerns (and some recommendations) but overall indicating that things are okay. I will read this twice a day until I get the results.	80/100
9	Attend my follow-up appointment for my annual physical/check-up.	75/100
8	A couple of days before my appointment, drive to my primary care provider's office and sit in the waiting room for 20 minutes (I will not be seeing the doctor this time).	70/100
7	Call and make an appointment with my orthopedist for the recent pain in my shoulder.	65/100
6	Call and make an appointment with my primary care provider for my annual physical/check-up.	60/100
5	Go to a random hospital and walk around for 1 hour. Visit various floors, waiting rooms, the cafeteria, etc. Will simply observe as I walk around.	55/100

Table 11 (*Continued*)

4	Go to a random urgent care or doctor office and sit in the waiting room for 30 minutes. Simply observe my environment.	**50/100**
3	Watch a show or movie that depicts various medical scenes or is set in a medical environment. If I have trouble watching it, I will watch it a second time a day or two later.	**45/100**
2	Imagine myself making an appointment with the orthopedist to inquire about the pain in my shoulder (i.e. imagine myself calling, the phone ringing, the receptionist asking for my information and reason for the appointment, me explaining my concerns, looking at the calendar, deciding on a date and then marking my calendar).	**40/100**
1	Imagine myself making an appointment with my primary care provider for my annual physical/check-up (i.e. imagine myself calling, the phone ringing, speaking with the receptionist, looking at the calendar, deciding on a date and then marking my calendar).	**40/100**

In Chapter 6 on page 147, I provided detailed tips for designing and implementing the exposure hierarchy, which are abbreviated here. Please make sure to complete your exposure planning log as well as your exposure experience log after each exposure exercise. These steps and tips are important to adhere to in order to maximize the benefits of using a fear hierarchy.

Tips for designing an exposure hierarchy

- Generalization is important in an exposure hierarchy.
- You can break up difficult tasks into smaller, manageable tasks.
- Safety behaviors can slowly be removed as you work your way up the hierarchy.
- Be vivid and specific with your imaginal exposure tasks.
- After completing your exposure hierarchy, you may want to design a new one.

Tips for completing tasks in an exposure hierarchy

- Prioritize your planning log.
- Try to accept and tolerate the anxiety during the exposure tasks.

- Use your adaptive coping techniques when exposure tasks get tough.
- Consider Socratic dialogue to be your best friend during exposures.
- Review imaginal exposures multiple times.
- Prioritize your exposure experience log.

References

1 Brady RE, Braz AN. Challenging interactions between patients with severe health anxiety and the healthcare system: A qualitative investigation. *Journal of Primary Care & Community Health.* 2023;14. <https://doi.org/10.1177/21501319231214876>

2 McBain S, Cordova MJ. Medical traumatic stress: Integrating evidence-based clinical applications from health and trauma psychology. *Journal of Traumatic Stress.* Published online July 6, 2024. <https://doi.org/10.1002/jts.23075>

3 Kazak AE, Kassam-Adams N, Schneider S, Zelikovsky N, Alderfer MA, Rourke M. An integrative model of pediatric medical traumatic stress. *Journal of Pediatric Psychology.* 2005;31(4):343–355. <https://doi.org/10.1093/jpepsy/jsj054>

4 Hall MF, Hall SE. *Managing the Psychological Impact of Medical Trauma: A Guide for Mental Health and Health Care Professionals.* Springer Publishing Company; 2017.

5 Sheynin J, Shind C, Radell M, et al. Greater avoidance behavior in individuals with posttraumatic stress disorder symptoms. *Stress.* 2017;20(3):285–293. <https://doi.org/10.1080/10253890.2017.1309523>

6 Kannan VD, Veazie PJ. Predictors of avoiding medical care and reasons for avoidance behavior. *Medical Care.* 2014;52(4):336–345.<https://doi.org/10.1097/mlr.0000000000000100>

7 Gómez de La Cuesta G, Schweizer S, Diehle J, Young J, Meiser-Stedman R. The relationship between maladaptive appraisals and posttraumatic stress disorder: A meta-analysis. *European Journal of Psychotraumatology.* 2019;10(1):1620084. <https://doi.org/10.1080/20008198.2019.1620084>

8 Horenstein A, Heimberg RG. Anxiety disorders and healthcare utilization: A systematic review. *Clinical Psychology Review*. 2020;81:101894. <https://doi.org/10.1016/j.cpr.2020.101894>

9 Tyrer P, Tyrer H. Health anxiety: Detection and treatment. *BJPsych Advances.* 2018;24(1):66–72. <https://doi.org/10.1192/bja.2017.5>

10 Whole Person Health: What it is and why it's important. NCCIH. Published 2020. <https://www.nccih.nih.gov/health/whole-person-health-what-it-is-and-why-its-important>

11 Know when to go to the ER. <www.emergencyphysicians.org.> <https://www.emergencyphysicians.org/article/know-when-to-go/know-when-to-go-overview>

12 Brady RE, Braz AN. Challenging interactions between patients with severe health anxiety and the healthcare system: A qualitative investigation. *Journal of Primary Care & Community Health*. 2023;14. <https://doi.org/10.1177/21501319231214876>

13 Rastegar PJ, Langhinrichsen-Rohling J. Understanding college students' healthcare avoidance: From early maladaptive schemas, through healthcare institutional betrayal and betrayal trauma appraisal of worst healthcare experiences. *Healthcare*. 2024; 12(11):1126. <https://doi.org/10.3390/healthcare12111126>

9

Become less afraid of death

Death anxiety, or thanatophobia, has been shown to play a prominent role in a wide range of psychological disorders.[1] In the aftermath of the pandemic, fears around mortality and loss are more common now than ever before.[2,3] Although death anxiety is transdiagnostic and presents itself across a wide variety of disorders, it is a particularly salient feature of health anxiety. And this isn't exactly surprising. After all, aside from being a victim of violence or in an accident of some kind, the vast majority of deaths are due to illness-related causes, right? Thus, it makes logical sense that many people struggle with both health anxiety and death anxiety.

Now, most people don't relish the idea of their death, but they accept to some degree that death is an inevitable part of life and they, more or less, leave it at that. However, many people with health anxiety find that their fear of illness and disease stems, at least in part, from fears related to death and/or the dying process. Only relatively recently have researchers and clinicians started to tackle this issue in their understanding and treatment of health anxiety.

The bottom line is this: if we try to improve your health anxiety without tackling your fear of death, we are merely slapping the proverbial band aid on your wound. Researchers refer to this as the 'revolving door' problem. Essentially, if a client comes to me for help with health anxiety and I don't address their death anxiety in treatment, the problem will likely resurface and they will be back again for treatment at some point in the future.

What's the worst that can happen?

A key Socratic question used in CBT is, 'What is the worst that can happen?' Now, when used to challenge other types of anxious thoughts, this question can be a slam dunk in terms of reducing anxiety. It highlights the irrationality of the fear, particularly when the worst thing that can happen is you stutter during a speech or someone thinks your idea is stupid. With health anxiety, however, the answer to this question isn't so comforting. Because what is the worst that can happen when your health goes south? Uh, you die. And if death is your biggest fear, this only further reinforces your perceived need to ensure that you are as healthy as possible, even if it is just to keep this whole death business at bay a little longer.

You, me, my Uber driver last night and everyone else on the planet will all be dead at some point in the future. Therefore, the critical question isn't about the probability of your death happening but about the cost or 'badness' of your death when it inevitably does happen. And *that*, my friends, is what we will be exploring in this chapter. But before we start down that morbid road, I'd like you to reflect on something. Is death really so bad that it is worth living the rest of your life crippled by the fear of it, whether you live for one more month or 65 more years?

Acknowledging and reconsidering your fears

After giving it a bit of thought, I will assume the answer to that question is a hard *no*. You probably recognize that life is short and aspire to be able to live more in the moment but you can't seem to free yourself from this underlying fear of death. After all, if it were that simple, you would have done it by now and could be out frolicking with friends rather than reading this book.

Before we get started, I want to recognize the difficulty of conversations around death and dying. This isn't an easy topic for most people but especially those with health and death anxiety. Be patient with yourself while working through this chapter and give yourself space to process these topics. It might be helpful to read only one section at a time and/or process this content with a trusted person. And prepare yourself—this chapter might make you cry. Not because it is oh-so-good but because we will be openly discussing topics you likely have avoided until now.

Many of my clients become overwhelmingly anxious when I begin to initiate conversations around death and dying. Of course, as with anything, and true to the very nature of exposure therapy, this fear tends to lessen the more we talk about it. Death has not been an easy topic for me either. I remember talking about death with a friend one night at dinner and then crying the whole drive home because I was so devastated by the idea of leaving loved ones behind. Today, I can talk about it like it's Sunday's brunch plans.

Now, let's unpack this fear. In my practice experience, I have noticed some patterns in the fear of death. Generally speaking, my clients (and I) have feared death for several different reasons:

1 fears about the dying process
2 fears about leaving loved ones behind
3 fears about the 'final destination' or what happens to you after you die

One or more of these reasons might resonate with you. And no judgment if it's all three (it was for me). Every one of these reasons has had me hanging on for dear life at various points in my own journey. It is important to tailor cognitive and behavioral interventions to fit each of these different reasons for fearing death. But the overall goal is the same: to help you learn that death is likely not going to be as bad as you think it will be, whether your concern is for you or your loved ones.

Fear of the dying process

People who fear the dying process itself often imagine catastrophic scenarios, such as being in intense physical pain, feeling humiliated in front of others, burdening loved ones who are caring for them and/or causing loved ones to be in emotional pain. I certainly have no shortage of humiliating and shame-filled scenarios about being on my deathbed. In one, I am bedridden at home and on hospice, sucking my dinner out of a straw while my husband is having an affair with one of the hot nurses. In another, a bunch of my relatives are sitting around my hospital bed talking, when the buzzing sound of conversation fades out as everyone begins to notice that my adult diaper is leaking urine, which drips down the bedpost and onto my cousin's shoes.

My clients have also described a number of bleak death fantasies to me, from medical staff refusing to give more morphine to kill the pain (or giving too much to hasten their death) to their mother attempting suicide because the pain of losing her child is unbearable. Whether experienced myself or told to me by my clients, I do not have a shortage of unpleasant tales about the death and dying process.

This paints quite the morose picture of the dying process. But keep in mind that this is all fiction. People with anxiety tend to have cognitive biases. Future scenarios, including death scenarios, are perceived to be more catastrophic than they likely will be in reality.

Many people with health anxiety assume dying inevitably involves intense physical and emotional pain. But the very goal of palliative and hospice care is to reduce physical, emotional and spiritual suffering among people with serious disease through a patient-centered approach.[4] Research on palliative care interventions suggests that they improve symptom burden and/or quality of life among patients with a variety of diseases.[5,6,7] The availability of palliative care has grown steadily, as 72 percent of hospitals in the United States with 50 beds or more and 90 percent of hospitals with 300 beds or more have palliative care teams.[8]

Rather ironically, despite my lifelong fear of death, I spent several years surrounded by it as a clinical social worker in hospice and hospital settings. I've worked with hundreds of dying patients and witnessed dozens of patient deaths. I have had the privilege of being able to provide comfort, support and direction to these patients and their families through the dying process. Through these experiences, I have seen large teams of medical, mental health and spiritual experts collaborate to promote patients' emotional and physical comfort.

The patients I worked with amazed me with their resilience, strength and determination. Many of them, just weeks or even days before death, were having intimate conversations with family and friends, laughing, making jokes, watching their favorite TV shows, eating junk food and even drinking their favorite beer. Sure, I was with my patients during some intensely hard moments. But they also shared a lot of meaningful moments with family, friends and their wider support system. Moments of anticipatory grief, regrets, anxiety and heartbreak were interwoven with reflection, vulnerability, honesty, reconciliation, support, gratitude, acceptance and even joy.

In addition to overestimating the pain and misery involved in death, people with health anxiety often assume that dying inevitably means that loved ones will be burdened by caring for them, resentful and/or inconsolable and unable to cope with the process of losing them. By catastrophizing or engaging in all-or-nothing thinking errors, we assume that if a loved one struggles, they will surely collapse and face utter ruin. Indeed, grief, caregiver burden and other difficult experiences related to losing a loved one are common and even expected. But personal characteristics, resources and support systems all play a vital role in how one copes with adversity.

During the years I worked with terminally ill patients, I spent an exorbitant amount of time with their family members and friends. I provided therapeutic support to help them manage their emotional pain, facilitated end-of-life decision-making processes and connected them to legal, medical, social and financial resources.

Through all of these experiences, do you know what stands out in my mind? Not the sadness or exhaustion, even though those were certainly present. But the incredible strength, resilience, commitment and determination exhibited by patients' loved ones just blew my mind. Loved ones showed up for the patient and for each other. Family members and friends drove or flew in from long distances, stayed up for days, made each other meals and comforted each other.

In addition, a key priority of hospice and palliative care is to ensure that the needs of loved ones are met. Our teams toiled collaboratively to support, encourage and guide loved ones through this difficult period. And this wasn't just my anecdotal experience. Research highlights the benefit of palliative and hospice care in reducing caregiver burden, financial costs, anxiety, depression and grief.[5,6,7,9]

So, what can we conclude from all of this? It is possible that how you have envisioned the dying process is based on biased and inaccurate assumptions. Of course, as is true with anything in life, we cannot be guaranteed a pleasant death. Unfortunate circumstances surrounding how one dies are possible. But it is likely that your death will not be as painful, terrifying or depressing as you fear it will be (and even if it is, it is short-term, with a definite end point). Nonetheless, with the support of family, friends, faith, pain management and other palliative care interventions as well as personal strength and resilience, there is sound reason to assume that you and your loved ones will be able to cope with this difficult process.

However, this information is not going to be nearly as helpful as it would be if you were to challenge your own assumptions. Below are some questions for you to consider, inspired by the type of Socratic dialogue used in CBT.

Table 1 Socratic questions to reconsider assumptions about the dying process

Fears around being humiliated during the final stages of a disease:
• Have you ever been with someone you loved during the dying process? Did you (or would you) think they should be ashamed or humiliated by relying on others? • What sorts of things would you do to help ensure someone close to you was able to maintain dignity while they were dying? How do you think your loved ones would do this for you? • In the past, have loved ones been okay with helping you in a time of need? Even if it meant having to rearrange plans, spend money and/or be inconvenienced in some way? Do you think, if you were dying, they might be even more willing to do this?
Fears around not wanting to be a burden to others during the dying process:
• Other than seeing you as a burden, how else might your loved ones see the opportunity to care for you? How would you see having to care for a loved one? • Even if your loved ones did experience caregiver burnout at some point, a very common experience, does that mean they don't want to care for you or don't love you? If you were exhausted from caring for a loved one, would this mean you didn't want to care for them or that you just needed some respite/recharge time? • How might your loved ones access additional support to cope with the demands of caring for you? Close family, extended relatives, friends, members of religious or other types of communities, hired help, palliative care professionals?
Fears around being in emotional or physical pain:
• How do you think palliative/hospice care might help you with physical pain? • In addition to all of your loved ones, what type of support would you want? Leaders of your religious organization to provide spiritual support or guidance and pray with you? Therapists/counselors/social workers? Other types of support? • What sorts of hobbies would make you feel stimulated, excited, entertained? Would you want your friends or family to be a part of any of these sorts of activities with you?

Imagine you are dying

Denial and avoidance of death-related concepts only increases the fear of it. As a society, in the USA and other westernized societies, we are guilty of promoting the avoidance of death and dying.[10] We do not embrace or openly talk about death in western culture. In fact, there has been a whole movement against this, sometimes referred to as 'death positivity,' which has advocated for greater acceptance of death in our culture by encouraging people to speak openly about death and dying.[11,12]

For example, people have death dinner parties to discuss mortality (e.g. acknowledging, understanding and talking about death-related fears, what people want and organizing or planning for death). Over 100,000 people have participated in these dinner parties around the globe.[13] In some ways, this 'death positivity' movement lends well to the basic tenets behind exposure therapy, which is to expose yourself to the feared stimulus to learn that it is not as terrifying as you assume.

One helpful first step toward exposing yourself to the concept of death is to use imaginal exposure. I often have my clients imagine themselves dying to become more comfortable with the dying process. To use myself as an example, the scariest movie I ever saw was *The Ring*. I was terrorized by images from the movie. I had nightmares and could not even stand to be alone for five minutes. And, because the excitement of it all got the best of me, I watched this movie again three or four more times over the next couple of weeks. However, each time I saw it, the movie had less and less of an impact. Consider the scariest movie you ever saw. Do you think you would be as terrified the 7th or the 15th time you saw it?

Similarly, the more you allow yourself to think about the dying process, the more you normalize it. Remember, no one expects you to revel in images of your death. We just want you to remove some of the fear that is preventing you from enjoying life. So, let me tell you a little story about my own death.

Table 2 An imaginal exposure exercise of my death

I am on hospice and laying on the hospital bed in my living room. Tubes around me, a hospice nurse sitting at my bedside. She is very kind and smells nice, like fresh soap. Her voice is always soothing. She keeps asking me if I am comfortable, making sure to adjust my medication as necessary to ensure I am not in any pain. Despite the progression of my disease, I am still alert and myself for the most part. Aside from bouts of exhaustion and discomfort, I can sit up and interact. My husband, Don, is having a conversation with our church pastor. My four-year-old son is moving around the room with his Paw Patrol truck, engaging with everyone, not completely aware of what is happening and as content as can be. My six-year-old daughter is sitting on the couch, laughing and asking questions as one of my best friends reads a book to her.

Table 2 (*Continued*)

The dining room table is pushed up against the wall and filled with a vivid, colorful display of fruits, vegetables, cheeses, sandwiches, appetizers, desserts, a big bucket of soft drinks and water bottles. Flower arrangements are placed throughout the room, infusing it with color. The front door is propped open because friends, family, neighbors, colleagues and church members are perpetually floating in and out, bringing flowers, food, candles, coffee, wine and presents for my son and daughter. The room is filled with the aroma of pumpkin-scented candles and the continual sound of scenes from *The Office*, *Friends* and *How I Met Your Mother* playing in the background.
Each day is filled with a different expression of love from the people in my life. On a couple of nights, a few of my close friends bring over rom-coms, junk food and wine. Some nights some friends and family come over just to pray with me, which brings me unspeakable peace and comfort. Other nights I spend just with Don and my kids, soaking up every minute with them and recording videos together. These moments in particular bring deep sadness but I am relieved by the joy of knowing that these videos will be invaluable to my children when they are older.
And then every once in a while, when everyone happens to be doing something, there is quiet. I sit in reflection, praying and thinking. Sometimes it feels scary and sad, other times I am overwhelmed by the love of God.
One day everyone comes together to give me a party, a celebration of life. We watch a video they all put together of me, that includes video clips and pictures, with some of my favorite bands playing in the background. We eat, laugh and my friends and family share some of their favorite stories about me. By the end of it, I feel more loved than I ever have before.
Several weeks pass by. Based on the progression of my symptoms, such as sleeping more, taking in less food and fluids, confusion and breathing changes, I might only have a few days left. I am continually fading in and out of sleep. Sensations of warmth come from a mixture of familiar voices and warm hands, then blackness again as I descend into a prolonged period of deep sleep and then back up again. Each wake period is met with different scenes of increasing brevity. At times my siblings, my best friends, Lynda or one of my aunts are sitting nearby conversing quietly while holding my hand, sometimes a nurse is feeding me ice chips, sometimes Don is sitting on the edge of my bed watching me, other times various people are clustered together in different parts of the room, talking or praying. My beautiful children are always busy little bees, moving about in the living room, often getting fed, praised and cuddled by everyone. Eventually, I stop being able to comprehend things. I just hear voices, see lights at times, but am mostly unaware. And then at one point, I close my eyes a final time and sink into the black.

This story was difficult for me to write. It is not a fun topic. But writing it out lessened some of my fears about the dying process specifically. I realized that in the bleak images of death that periodically flashed through my mind, I was only acknowledging the depressing, scary parts and not any of the beauty—the support, kindness, love and comfort. In addition, some of the scariest parts for me, such as slowly becoming less and less like myself as the disease progresses and the final moment when I draw my last breath, didn't seem nearly as bad once I wrote down these feared scenarios.

Now, do I know my death will turn out this way? Of course not. It is possible that the nurse is rude and smells like cigarette smoke, my family and friends are angry and arguing with each other and I am in pain and no one is listening to me as I beg them to up my morphine drip. All of this *could* happen but is it likely to happen? No. It is likely that my final weeks, days and moments will be filled with love, support and comfort, even in the presence of all the challenges. And even when I do experience physical pain, discomfort and unpleasant emotions, it won't be continuous. It will fluctuate and have an endpoint.

I can say this confidently because I know my family and friends and, having worked in hospice for several years, I also know how caring the hospice teams are likely to be. Remember, research shows that anxiety leads people to catastrophize future situations. The 'good parts' in my dying experience might look very different from the ones I have envisioned in my imaginal exposure exercise. But, no doubt, there will be beauty and comfort mixed in there. And it is also possible that my experience will be even better than I described.

Now, it's your turn. Let's get those creative juices flowing. I'd like you to write out your own death narrative. A couple of tips to consider before you get started.

- **Don't think about what your experience should be but what you actually want it to be.** We are all unique. For me, having multiple people float in and out of my house to spend time with me before I die is exactly what would bring me joy. For you, that may sound like hell. Make it work for you. In real life you and/or your family will be creating this scenario to some extent, of course barring situations like a sudden death or rapid decline. We want this exposure exercise to be as close to reality as possible and to capture you and what you are comfortable with.

- **Make your story as vivid and specific as possible.** You will not connect with your story if you write some vague, overgeneralized story such as you go to the hospital, hug everyone and then die. No, imaginal exposure is much more effective the more believable it is. And that means getting real with it. One helpful technique is to start by making a list of both what you would want as well as the most likely elements of your death situation.

Write out your story. After you are done, record it and listen to it two to three times a day for one week. The first time I wrote out my death scene, everything about it felt gross. I even got choked up when I wrote about my children playing near my hospital bed. But after listening to it multiple times a day for a period of time, the images from my story, and the idea of my death in general, grew less and less intimidating. Eventually, I got about as worked up as I do when I read my grocery store list.

In-vivo exposure exercises to face fears of the dying process

Death anxiety, just like health anxiety, can lead us to avoid anything that makes us think of it. Thus, naturally, one helpful way to improve death anxiety is to systematically expose yourself to reminders of death. Essentially, you want to grow more comfortable with the idea of death over time.

We introduced in-vivo exposures in Chapter 6. Below are a few in-vivo exposure exercises to reduce anxiety over the dying process. Keep in mind that we are all unique and different exposure tasks work better for some than others. You may need to tweak your exposure tasks to better fit you. Review the steps and tips for implementing exposure hierarchies on page 148 to refresh your memory on how to successfully implement exposure tasks. Keep in mind that the goal of exposure exercises is to help you to grow more comfortable and accepting of the idea of death and dying.

Table 3 Exposure exercises to face the fear of the dying process

- Watch movies or read fiction books with scenes of people dying
- Review hospice materials—many of them talk about the dying process in detail
- Read about people who have lost loved ones and have cared for them during the dying process or memoirs written by people who are dying
- Develop a plan for how you would like your dying process to be if you were able to choose. Where would you be (e.g. in hospital, at home or at a relative's under hospice care), who would be there, what food and drink would you want to enjoy and what sorts of activities would you like to do, depending on your energy/comfort level (play games, watch shows, listen to music, visit with loved ones)?
- Write down the special things you imagine your loved ones would say to you if you were dying in the hospital or at home under hospice care
- Read about death dinners (deathoverdinner.org)
- Attend a death dinner and share about how you would like to die if you died from an illness-related cause
- Visit a cemetery—take a nice, long walk through the cemetery, reading the headstones. Try to imagine the lives of these people on these headstones and what the dying process was like for them.

Fear of leaving loved ones behind

Many of the health-anxious clients I've worked with come to realize that their death anxiety stems from the fear of leaving their children behind. The concern about a child's well-being after losing a parent isn't a minor concern that can be easily dismissed. For example, it is arguably harder to challenge anxious thoughts about whether your kids will be okay after you die than it is to challenge thoughts about what other people think. As a mother of young children, I have asked all of these questions and faced these fears myself. In this section, I am going to specifically address the fear of leaving children behind. However, note that you can apply these concepts to the fear of leaving any loved ones behind, such as your partner, parents, siblings or other relatives or friends.

The fear that your child would not be okay if you were to die is *understandable*. But this doesn't mean all of the assumptions you are making about their well-being after your death are valid. By assuming your children or other loved ones would not be able to thrive without you, you are likely underestimating their ability to cope with losing you. There is a wide variety of factors that contribute to a person's well-being. Maybe you are not accounting for many of the factors that would have a positive impact on your child's well-being, such as the love and support from a remaining parent, loved ones stepping in to care for your child and your child's personal strengths and resilience. As with any other type of anxiety, we must examine your thoughts, beliefs and underlying assumptions more closely.

My mother was always terrified that she would die because she did not think my brother and I would be okay without her. After all, my father was homeless and on drugs so he clearly was not going to swoop in and save the day. Because of her fear, my mom made arrangements. She purchased life insurance. She took her best friend, Lynda, and Lynda's husband, Duncan, out to dinner and formally asked them if they'd be willing to take us into their home should anything happen to her (to which they happily agreed). She also had conversations with me from time to time about taking care of my little brother if something ever happened to her.

As it turned out, my mother's worst fear did come true. She died suddenly from a pain medication overdose when I was 16 and my brother was 15. It was tragic. And suddenly the worst possible 'what-if' scenario was staring me right in the face. Many people, including my brother and I, were not okay in the days that followed November 28, 1996.

Yet there is so much more to this story. The shock, despair and fear my brother and I experienced were met with more comfort and support than I had ever encountered. And it wasn't just an outpouring of phone calls, visits, food, gifts and flowers that faded as soon as the funeral was over. People didn't just show up for us, they stuck around. My godparents, Lynda and Duncan, immediately drove up to Santa Cruz from Huntington Beach after she died. They were with us from the week after she died and up through today. All of our other relatives and friends have also stepped up in unique ways and played large roles in our lives.

It was prudent and wise for my mom to make arrangements in the event of her death. Given that she had health issues, and we did not have another viable parent to take over, it was necessary to take reasonable steps to ensure our safety and well-being.

However, it was unnecessary for her to spend years worrying excessively about an endless number of potential negative outcomes.

Despite the irreparable loss of a mother, we turned out fine. We both struggled in various ways, but we mostly turned out okay. And there are many identifiable reasons for this, such as spiritual faith, support from loved ones and personal strength and resilience.

Just like my mom, your assumptions about your child's well-being in the event of your death may not be completely accurate. Just like we've done with other anxious thoughts about your health, it can be helpful to formally examine the evidence for these thoughts.

Examine the evidence

Let's briefly review the details of this activity that we introduced in Chapter 3. Write down a specific thought about your child or loved one's well-being if you were to die. On a scale of 1–100, document the degree to which you believe this thought (1 indicating very little, 100 indicating very strong). We begin by documenting all of the evidence *in support* of the thought or belief. Note that it is important that you include all of the reasons, no matter how silly it seems. You need to bring it out in the open so you can challenge it. Otherwise, it remains in the back of your head as 'evidence' and will continue to reinforce this view. We then write down all of the evidence *against* the thought or belief.

Afterward, it is important to go back and review the evidence in *support* of the belief and challenge any potentially distorted thoughts. As we know, with anxiety we tend to be biased in our thinking so it is critical to ensure that we challenge any items that you have mentally logged as 'evidence' for the thought that aren't necessarily accurate.

Once you are finished, review all of the evidence. Sit with it for a bit. Then reassess the degree to which you believe the thought on a scale of 1–100. This will help you see if the activity had any impact. Note, even if the strength of your belief is only reduced by a few points, I would consider that a success. It would be unreasonable to think that you would drop to 0 or anything close to that. Reshaping thoughts about beliefs happens slowly as you continue to do this work on a consistent basis.

Examine the Evidence

Anxious thought: Ariel and Erick will not be okay without me.

Degree of belief before the exercise (0–100): **85/100**

Evidence FOR the thought

- If I die, Ariel and Erick will be without the comfort of a mother. *REFRAME: Yes, they would not have the comfort from me that they are used to. But there are many people in their lives that can, at least partially, fill this maternal role. They will also have the security of knowing how much I loved them.*
- I am the sensitive and compassionate parent and my spouse, Jim, can be harsh/strict in his parenting style. *REFRAME: Jim is not naturally compassionate/sensitive but he is aware of it and has improved over the years. Plus, there will be plenty of other family/friends that are soft spoken and compassionate, such as my mom, siblings, friends, and in-laws.*
- I am the parent who adds the sparkle to holidays, special occasions and events (e.g. plans everything around holidays, birthdays, kid parties). There will inevitably be less 'sparkle' without me around. *REFRAME: Yes, there might be less 'sparkle' in some ways. But Jim knows I love doing these types of activities and would definitely step in to do more of this if he needed to. Plus my mother-in-law is really good at this stuff too. She, and others, would put in a lot of effort to make holidays and other events special in my absence). Also, even if there is less 'sparkle' my kids will still be okay. They will be loved and that is most important.*
- I handle everything kid-related (e.g. school prep, packing lunches, field trips). My kids won't have as much support in these little ways if I'm not here. *REFRAME: Jim and relatives would step up and do what needs to be done. Even if they miss something, these are minor things and my kids will be okay, even without all of this. Plus, there are likely small ways they gain in some way that I can't even think of. My sister-in-law does special little extra things for her kids that I don't do. She may even do some of that for my kids. It is impossible to know and weigh all the details. Regardless, these things won't make or break them.*

- Have come across information about the struggle a child goes through after the loss of a parent (e.g. in my social circles, in non-fiction books and movies based on real-life stories). *REFRAME: Of course they would struggle if I died. However, this isn't a permanent state. They would grow. The research shows that people can thrive and become stronger after adversity/trauma. My mom grew up without a dad and she struggled at times but ultimately had a great life.*
- My father grew up with one parent and he struggled. *REFRAME: He struggled but he turned out okay. What's more, even his one remaining parent had a lot of issues and he still turned out okay. Ariel and Erick are already way more fortunate than my dad ever was.*

Evidence AGAINST the thought

- Ariel and Erick will have a ton of other people around to help take care of them and to love them, including my mom, sisters, best friend and my husband's family as well as cousins and neighborhood friends: a small but mighty community.
- My kids have a ton of memories of me loving and caring for them. They have thousands of videos, pictures, letters, cards that show how much I loved them, even when they forget or the memories fade. They will always know that their mother loved them more than anything in the world.
- I have a life insurance policy. If I died, Jim and the kids would have a little extra money to put away for the kids' college and to provide a little childcare.
- Even though my kids would, of course, be devastated if they lost me, they would continue on. They will still be alive and enjoy all of the wonderful things life has to offer. They will play, learn, make friends, enjoy school, win sports games, go to prom, maybe go to college, get married, have an amazing career, travel, and/or have kids of their own.
- I have known lots of people (friends, family) who grew up with only one parent because of abandonment, divorce or death. All of

these people are doing okay. One of my friends even lost her dad in a car accident when she was younger and it was very traumatic. And yet, she is doing really well right now.

- Jim is a good father and loves our kids. He is protective and cares for them. He would always have their best interest in mind.
- Human resilience is an amazing thing. Many people have survived and even thrived after a lot of traumatic life events. Likewise, my kids would grow from this very difficult experience and could be stronger and better people. For example, they might be more mindful of how precious life is and be able to live more in the present moment. Or they might be more compassionate with others because they've been through a very painful experience themselves.
- My kids have grown up with love and in a healthy environment. They already know they are loved and are secure because of it. This would contribute to their resilience and would help them cope with losing me.

Degree of belief after the exercise (0–100): **45/100**

As you've read many times, we often don't realize how flawed our assumptions can be. It can be helpful to pull back and take a 'bird's eye view' and to see all of your thoughts together in one place. This exercise was a pivotal step for me in reconsidering my own assumptions about leaving my children behind. I realized that what I originally perceived to be evidence for the thought that my children would not be okay was not necessarily valid. I also hadn't considered many of the reasons why my kids would still be able to thrive and enjoy life even in my absence. It allowed me to take a step back, evaluate everything and develop a more balanced view.

Notably, things do not happen in a vacuum. Losing a parent would not be your children's only experience, nor would it be their sole identity. In fact, decades of research in developmental psychology underscore that multiple risk and protective factors across multiple systems influence developmental pathways for children.[14] Essentially, two children could go through the same experience and be impacted in very different ways depending on many other risk and protective factors, a concept known as multifinality.[15] All of this is to say that a child's 'well-being' does not rest on any one particular variable, such as the experience of losing a parent.

More broadly, consider the large body of research on human resilience and post-traumatic growth, suggesting that traumatic experiences can be a 'catalyst' for positive change. Specifically, traumatic experiences can lead to improved relationships and new life possibilities as well as an increase in self-awareness, personal strengths, appreciation for life and spiritual development.[16,17,18,19,20] There is plenty of evidence to suggest that hardship can make us stronger and more resilient.

I know that losing my mother at an early age prompted change and growth in a number of ways. I had a renewed sense of interest in my faith as well as a lot more empathy and compassion for others. I also become incredibly grateful for my loved ones. I dedicated way more energy and time to staying closely connected with my family and friends. In addition, prior to my mom dying, I had become a rather lazy and irresponsible student. In the couple of years that followed her death, I transformed into a laser-focused, dedicated student and eventually got into UCLA. Looking back, not having my mother challenged me to become a more loving, dedicated, curious and driven person.

Reconsidering assumptions about your loved ones' well-being

Similarly, it can be helpful to consider all the reasons your children might be just fine and even thrive if you were to die. We anxious folk are so good at using our imaginations to dream up all the ways things can go terribly wrong. Isn't it fair, then, to also consider how things might go well? (1) think through the reasons *why* your children might be okay (e.g. personal strengths, resources, support network) if they were to lose you; as well as (2) imagine the ways your child might be able to grow, evolve and enjoy a good life after facing the challenge of losing you. Below are a few questions you can use to inspire a new way of thinking about this.

Table 4 Socratic questions about loved ones' well-being after your death

Recognizing the power of personal strengths and resilience:
• Considering the powerful potential of human resilience, what types of hard things have you been through and in what ways did these things give way to personal growth and strengthening? • What types of trauma or adversity have your children or other loved ones been through? How have they been able to cope? How have they been able to heal and grow from this? • Do you think it is plausible that the people in your life would be able to cope with the heartbreak of losing you? How so? • How do you think your relationship with your loved ones and what they have gained or learned from you might help them cope with the loss of you? Think of all the ways you have poured into them—building their self-confidence and self-esteem, helping them to know they are lovable, valuable and worthy. Think of how you show up for them, offering a consistent, reliable, trustworthy presence. • Consider your loved ones' individual strengths. What are they good at? Where and in what ways do they thrive? How have they impressed you or surprised you? • How might losing you lead to your children or other loved ones experiencing some of the positive outcomes in the post-traumatic growth research (e.g. development of new strengths and greater self-awareness, new opportunities, greater appreciation for life, increased spiritual development)? Can you try to envision some of this happening? How would it manifest in your children's or other loved ones' lives?
Recognizing other resources:
Social resources • Who will step in to care for your children (or if you have a partner, who will step in to help your partner care for them)? Consider who will be their primary caregivers but also consider all of the additional people that will be in their lives and provide love and support. This could be relatives, friends, neighbors, members of a church or other religious community, colleagues, or people in your children's school or extracurricular community. • How do you think these loved ones will keep your memory alive and ensure that your children will know about you and how much you loved them? For example, will they tell stories, show pictures and videos, share things about you and the things you did or how you lived your life? How will they continue to foster the values and priorities that are important to you? For example, religion and spirituality, education, hobbies, kindness and caring for others, relationships, work ethic. **Religious/spiritual resources** • How might your children's religion/faith/spirituality/cultural traditions provide support in the midst of enduring the loss of you? What are some of the key tenets of this religion, faith, spiritual path or cultural traditions that might help them cope with their grief/loss?

- Is there a community they belong to that would continue to provide support? In what ways would they provide support? Can you picture how this might play out in their daily, weekly or monthly lives?

Financial resources

- Do you have any financial resources that might offer additional support/help? For example, do you have savings that your partner or family members who are caring for your children can draw from for additional support?
- Do you have a life insurance policy? Do you have a will in place? How might one or two of these things offer additional support to your children and loved ones after you pass?
- If you are limited in financial resources, is it possible that your loved ones might be able to access additional help via GoFundMe campaigns or help from relatives, friends or the church community?

Mental health resources

- How might additional support services provide help to your children to cope with grief and loss, such as support groups, individual therapy, family therapy, group counseling? Consider the cheap or free resources that are available at schools, in the community, through non-profits or in churches and other faith-based organizations.

In-vivo exposure exercises to face the fear of leaving loved ones behind

As stated earlier, one evidence-based technique for improving the fear of death is to systematically expose yourself to death-related concepts or reminders. When targeting specific death-related fears, such as the fear of leaving loved ones behind, it can be helpful to tailor exposure exercises to face that specific fear. I don't expect you to ever relish the idea of leaving loved ones behind, of course. I just want you to get to a place in which you can accept it as a normal part of life and not live in fear of it.

Again, review the steps and tips for implementing exposure hierarchies on page 148 to refresh your memory on how to successfully implement exposure tasks. Keep in mind that the goal of exposure exercises is to help you to grow more comfortable and accepting of the idea of death and dying.

Managing and adaptively coping with anxiety involves taking reasonable or practical steps to address an issue and then practicing acceptance and letting go beyond those reasonable steps. In the context of fears around leaving loved ones behind, there may be practical steps you want to take to plan for your death (of course, only steps that are in your control). You could put together a will, make arrangements with those you wish to care for your kids should you unexpectedly die and/or get a life insurance policy. Thus, these exposure tasks can provide the dual benefit of helping you grow more comfortable with the idea of your death as well as helping you take practical steps to plan for your children. For me, putting together a will and getting a life insurance policy reduced my anxiety because I knew I had done what was in my control to promote their well-being in the event of my death.

Table 5 Exposure tasks to face the fear of leaving loved ones behind

- Watch movies, shows or read books about children who lost a parent when they were a child or young adult. Reflect on the positives about the stories; how did their characters cope, grow or learn?
- Create a will for your children and meet with a lawyer to put plans in place (might include writing letters to children and loved ones that will be caring for them, details about how finances are delegated and by whom, estate planning)
- Purchase a life insurance policy and/or come up with a financial plan to help support your children/other loved ones if you were gone
- Talk to your spouse/their other parent about what is most important to you regarding how the children would be cared for after you die (e.g. they remain a part of a religious community, reside geographically close to family, their education is prioritized, they remain in the same schools)
- Meet with the person/people who will care for your children if you (and your spouse/any other parent) are no longer around. Talk to them about the specifics of what is important to you
- Attend a death dinner (deathoverdinner.org) and share about what you would want for your children or other loved ones if you were to die
- Write letters to be given to your children in the event of your death (could just be letters for the purposes of this exercise and never given to your children or could be included in the will to be given to your children (some people have one letter or you could have more than one letter that will be given to them based on children's age/life stage)
- Record video or audio clips for your children to have after you die (and store them somewhere safe like a Google Drive or external hard drive)
- Conduct an imaginal exposure exercise. Write, type or audio record a story about your kids living life after you are gone. Write the details as the years go on, such as the things they will be doing and their successes and challenges. When facing challenges, write about their strengths, resilience and support system—imagine the ways they will be resilient and cope well in the months and years after you are gone. Imagine how they will thrive. Listen or read to this script at least once a day for a week

Fear of the 'Final Destination'

Some people have death anxiety because they worry about where they will go when they die. They worry about not existing anymore or whether they will be damned to hell, purgatory or some other 'non-heavenly' place. These uncertainties are certainly complex. We all have our ideas, beliefs, theories and, in one way or another, we put our faith into these various things. However, at the end of the day, until we die we can't be certain. Still, it is likely that some of your fears are based on unhelpful assumptions. Let's explore them because you might be overestimating just how terrible things will be for you after you die.

First, let's briefly discuss anxiety over being damned to hell or some other non-paradise. Why, according to the tenets of your faith, do you believe you have earned hell-status? Recall that if you have anxiety, you tend to overestimate threats in your environment, which colors how you interpret situations. Is it possible that you have exaggerated the 'threat' in this situation too?

Often what I've observed from my clients is that their beliefs about hell are not necessarily aligned with the theological underpinnings of their religion. I know for me, personally, growing up in a Christian household, I spent years living in fear of going to hell. Delightful images regularly splashed across my mind of me burning in a lake of fire, which most certainly contributed to my fear of death. But eventually I came to terms with the discrepancy between my assumptions and Christian theology. Actually, my husband's expertise in theology, from the Master of Divinity he earned at Princeton University, helped me grapple with these fears. To that end, for these types of concerns, it may be helpful for you to speak with a spiritual adviser within your religious community who can sufficiently answer these types of questions.

Now, let's discuss worries about not existing anymore. Of course, the idea of not existing is disconcerting. How could it not be? We experience all the joys and pains of life and everything in between. We love, suffer, fail, thrive and learn and grow in countless ways. And for what? To just close our eyes one day and succumb to nothingness. The idea of this is not exactly thrilling and rather sad. Because the reality is, other than those who are in unbearable emotional or physical pain, we all want to live. The point here is that it is perfectly natural to want to remain a conscious, living being.

If it is, indeed, true that there is no God or afterlife and all religion is just seeking immortality in vain, then, quite frankly, we have no choice but to accept it. So why give up the enjoyment of the potentially dozens of years you have left by fighting it, fretting about it and even being terrorized by it?

Now, let's dissect the whole notion of dying and transitioning into nothingness. I'll start with a simple question. Will you ever know what it is like to not exist? Nope. Awareness is only possible when we are conscious. Right now, as living beings, we can try to imagine it. But after we draw that last breath, we aren't sitting around in the darkness thinking about how much it sucks to not exist. You didn't exist before you were born. Were you sad then, anxiously anticipating the day you were going to be born? No, you weren't, just like you aren't going to be looking back longingly at the life you once had. In a way, there are gifts that come with not being conscious.

Consider your nightly experience of falling asleep. You might notice when you begin to feel sleepy as you are reading a book, playing on your phone or staring into the dark room. But once you fall asleep, you aren't thinking, *oh I am so glad I am sleeping right now and getting rest*. You don't realize you fell asleep until you wake up again. If, indeed, there is no afterlife then when you die it is simply as if you fell asleep and never woke up again. You only have to endure the sadness or anxiety in the moments leading up to you 'falling asleep.' And then you are free.

As I mentioned earlier, I believe wholeheartedly that there is more to this life than what we see in our physical world. Consider me in the God, heaven, life-after-death 'camp.' But do I know this for *sure*? Of course not. I am not dead. I fully recognize the possibility that I am completely wrong about this. That we all merely become part of the Earth after we die and life and consciousness end when we draw our last breath. If this ends up being true then, oh well, I guess I'll never know! I won't even experience the grief that would accompany that reality because, having no consciousness, I won't actually be aware of it. Thinking of it this way has been freeing for me. Sure, I hope with all my heart that I am right. But there is certainly no pain involved if it turns out I am wrong.

Imagine yourself losing consciousness

Picture yourself closing your eyes for the last time. The act of drifting into a new physical state is not hard to imagine because we practice something similar when we fall asleep. Obviously, death is not the same in terms of the *outcome*. But the *process* is similar. If it is true that we don't exist once we die, then the actual outcome of not being alive anymore isn't going to affect you because you won't even know it. Only the process will affect you.

So let's practice the process! Think of the hundreds of thousands of times you have fallen asleep. Picture it over and over again. Starting to drift into a new state, losing recognition of your senses, fading ever so slowly, and then sinking into the dark void. That's not so bad is it? Practice this over and over for a week. Then do a check-in and see if the idea stings less, even if just in small ways.

Reconsidering assumptions about what happens after death

Again, it can be helpful to use critical thinking to explore your assumptions about what happens after death. As you well know by now, this can be done with Socratic dialogue. We want you to use logic and reasoning to critically evaluate some of your assumptions, dissect and flip these concepts around and develop new viewpoints. Below are a few questions to get you started. I encourage you to think of your own questions as well, as this will help you continue to sharpen your critical thinking skills.

Table 6 Socratic questions about your posthumous legacy and/or experience

- How will your loved ones ensure that your memory lives on even though you are gone? Through pictures of you, videos, things you have written or created?
- Think about your legacy or the impact you have had on the world, whether big or small. How will this live on even if you aren't alive anymore?
- Think about the impact you have had on all of your loved ones' lives. What would people say about you at your funeral? In what ways have you had a positive impact on your loved ones' lives? How will this impact continue to serve people even after you are gone?
- If you believe in God and an afterlife, what are some of the reasons you assume prove you deserve to go to hell? Is there any evidence against this? How might this be incongruent with the tenets of your religion? Is there an alternative way to view this?
- What are some reasons you might go to heaven to be with God? How are these reasons supported by your religion's texts and traditions?
- Thinking about the idea of no longer being conscious, can you come up with reasons why this wouldn't be as awful as you are expecting it to be? How can you make peace with this idea? Are there people you trust that you can initiate conversations about this with?

In-vivo exposure exercises to face the fear of what happens after death

Next, I'd like to help you face posthumous concepts and reminders through exposure exercises. When targeting specific death-related fears, such as the fear over what happens after death, it can be helpful to tailor exposure exercises to face that specific fear. Essentially, you want to grow more comfortable with the idea of dying and no longer being a part of this world. The goal is not to love the idea of death but just to not live in such fear of it that you can't enjoy the life you have right now. Review the steps and tips for implementing exposure hierarchies in Chapter 6 (on page 148) to refresh your memory on how to successfully implement exposure tasks.

Table 7 Exposure tasks to face the fear of what happens after death

- Read obituaries in the newspaper to see how memories live on with the loved ones of the deceased.
- Watch movies, shows or read fiction books about the afterlife (pick those that match up with your views, values, traditions, beliefs).
- Read books written by leaders of your religion about the afterlife.
- Read books written by agnostic or atheist authors who talk about the idea of not existing or no longer being conscious.
- If you are religious/spiritual/a person of faith, how can you reconnect with the appropriate organizations, communities, traditions?
- Write down what you would like your headstone to say after you die.
- Conduct an imaginal exposure exercise in which you imagine all of the things your loved ones would say at your funeral/memorial service or afterward at a gathering. Think through each of your closest loved ones and write down what they would say about how you have impacted their lives.
- Visit a cemetery and read all of the headstones. Picture your headstone as well and read aloud what you wrote about yourself on your imaginary headstone.
- Talk to leaders at your religious organization to discuss fears about not going to heaven.
- Go to a funeral home and lay in a casket if you are able to (or create a makeshift one at home). Close your eyes and lay still for a while. Imagine your body being lifeless.

References

1 Iverach L, Menzies RG, Menzies RE. Death anxiety and its role in psychopathology: Reviewing the status of a transdiagnostic construct. *Clinical Psychology Review.* 2014;34(7):580–593. <https://doi.org/10.1016/j.cpr.2014.09.002>

2 Patra I, Iskandar Muda, Ngakan Ketut Acwin Dwijendra, et al. A systematic review and meta-analysis on death anxiety during COVID-19 pandemic. *OMEGA – Journal of Death and Dying.* Published online June 29, 2023. <https://doi.org/10.1177/00302228221144791>

3 Muazzam A, Naseem F, Shakil M, Visvizi A, Klemens J. Surviving COVID-19: Biopsychosocial impacts, death anxiety, and coping strategies. *Vaccines.* 2023;11(3):705. <https://doi.org/10.3390/vaccines11030705>

4 National Institute on Aging. What are palliative care and hospice care? National Institute on Aging. Published May 14, 2021. <https://www.nia.nih.gov/health/hospice-and-palliative-care/what-are-palliative-care-and-hospice-care>

5 Kavalieratos D, Corbelli J, Zhang D, et al. Association between palliative care and patient and caregiver outcomes. *JAMA.* 2016;316(20):2104. <https://doi.org/10.1001/jama.2016.16840>

6 Sharafi S, Ziaee A, Dahmardeh H. What are the outcomes of hospice care for cancer patients? A systematic review. *Supportive Care in Cancer.* 2022;31(1). <https://doi.org/10.1007/s00520-022-07524-2>

7 Quinn KL, Shurrab M, Gitau K, et al. Association of receipt of palliative care interventions with health care use, quality of life, and symptom burden among adults with chronic noncancer illness. *JAMA.* 2020;324(14):1439. <https://doi.org/10.1001/jama.2020.14205>

8 Dumanovsky T, Augustin R, Rogers M, Lettang K, Meier DE, Morrison RS. The growth of palliative care in U.S. hospitals: A status report. *Journal of Palliative Medicine.* 2016;19(1):8–15. <https://doi.org/10.1089/jpm.2015.0351>

9 Currow DC, Agar MR, Phillips JL. Role of hospice care at the end of life for people with cancer. *Journal of Clinical Oncology.* 2020;38(9):JCO.18.02235. <https://doi.org/10.1200/jco.18.02235>

10 Gire J. How death imitates life: Cultural influences on conceptions of death and dying. *Online Readings in Psychology and Culture.* 2014;6(2). <https://doi.org/10.9707/2307-0919.1120>

11 Incorvaia AD. Death Positivity in America: The movement—its history and literature. *OMEGA – Journal of Death and Dying.* Published online April 23, 2022:003022282210851. <https://doi.org/10.1177/00302228221085176>

12 Death Positive Movement. The order of the good death. <https://www.orderofthegooddeath.com/death-positive-movement/>

13 Death over dinner. Death Over Dinner. Published 2019. <https://deathoverdinner.org>

14 Masten AS, Lucke CM, Nelson KM, Stallworthy IC. Resilience in development and psychopathology: Multisystem perspectives. *Annual Review of Clinical Psychology*. 2021;17(1). <https://doi.org/10.1146/annurev-clinpsy-081219-120307>

15 Cicchetti D, Rogosch FA. Equifinality and multifinality in developmental psychopathology. *Development and Psychopathology.* 1996;8(4):597–600. <https://doi.org/10.1017/s0954579400007318>

16 Henson C, Truchot D, Canevello A. What promotes post traumatic growth? A systematic review. *European Journal of Trauma & Dissociation.* 2020;5(4):100195. <https://doi.org/10.1016/j.ejtd.2020.100195>

17 Calhoun LG, Tedeschi RG, eds. *Handbook of Posttraumatic Growth.* Routledge; 2014. <https://doi.org/10.4324/9781315805597>

18 Tedeschi RG, Moore BA. Posttraumatic growth as an integrative therapeutic philosophy. *Journal of Psychotherapy Integration*. 2020;31(2):180–194. <https://doi.org/10.1037/int0000250>

19 Su YJ, Chen SH. Emerging posttraumatic growth: A prospective study with pre- and posttrauma psychological predictors. *Psychological Trauma: Theory, Research, Practice, and Policy.* 2015;7(2):103–111. <https://doi.org/10.1037/tra0000008>

20 Linley PA, Joseph S. Positive change following trauma and adversity: A review. *Journal of Traumatic Stress.* 2004;17(1):11–21. <https://doi.org/10.1023/b:jots.0000014671.27856.7e>

10

Improving health anxiety in the face of a real medical condition

Getting diagnosed with a medical condition can be destabilizing, disrupting one's overall sense of safety, comfort and predictability in life. Further, the physical, psychological and practical challenges of managing and coping with a disease can be a significant burden. One is forced to grapple with changes and challenges never faced before, such as the loss of certain parts of themselves or their life, fears about the future, symptom burden, diagnosis and treatment burden and financial concerns. Given these challenges, it is not surprising that people facing medical conditions can experience a surge in health anxiety and other forms of psychological distress.[1,2]

Although living with a medical condition can be incredibly challenging, it doesn't mean you inevitably must live with health anxiety for the rest of your life or for as long as you have this disease. By working on your anxiety, you can improve your quality of life no matter what type of disease you face or stage of disease you are in. Disease and debilitating anxiety are not synonymous. Please note that if you are struggling with a medical condition, all of the techniques taught in this book are relevant for you. It is important that you master the skills taught in all of the chapters up to this point. However, this chapter is intended to serve as an additional resource for those experiencing anxiety while facing a medical condition.

My client, who was in her early thirties, lived with both cancer and lung disease. Yes, she had her struggles and bad days. Life was far from perfect. Yet, she managed to still find joy. She was passionate about working toward her career goals. She loved knitting and proudly sold her pieces online. She enjoyed fashion and prioritized her weekly manicure. She reveled in her periodic crushes on guys she interacted with at work or at the hospital where she got her treatments. Essentially, despite her struggles and losses, she still found ways to be herself, live in a way that aligned with some of her core values and be present-focused. Through learning to reshape problematic thinking and behavior as well as building coping skills and self-efficacy, it is possible to reduce anxiety over your health struggles and improve quality of life.

How illness-related beliefs impact daily life

Throughout this book, we have discussed common core belief themes experienced by those with health anxiety (e.g. beliefs about weakness or susceptibility, disease, uncertainty, death, medicine) as well as the impact of these beliefs on daily experiences. In that same vein, research suggests that we develop illness-related beliefs throughout life and during the course of an illness.[3] Essentially, when one faces a medical condition, they draw on their understanding of health threats, which is derived from both experiences prior to diagnosis as well as experiences during the course of the disease. These beliefs guide emotional and behavioral responses to the disease.[4]

Like all beliefs, some of these might be adaptive and helpful while others might be maladaptive and less helpful. Adaptive illness-related beliefs are conceptualized as *facilitating* beliefs and increase one's ability to identify adaptive solutions, manage the illness and reduce suffering.[5,6] Contrarily, *constraining* illness-related beliefs can promote more problems, restrict options and increase suffering.[5,6] It is, therefore, crucial to reshape constraining beliefs into facilitating beliefs, which will, in turn, lead to more adaptive thoughts and behaviors in one's day-to-day experience and improve overall functioning and emotional well-being in the face of a medical condition.

The cycle of health anxiety with a medical condition

Getting diagnosed with and managing a medical condition can, understandably, trigger anxiety related to fears of the future. Perhaps you have already struggled with health anxiety and it has been exacerbated as your biggest fear is staring you right in the face. Or maybe dealing with health anxiety is a new experience for you, prompted by the health challenges you are now facing. Regardless, new and scary fears are turning up that you may never have experienced before, such as:

- health outcomes or recurrence
- career loss or changes
- financial burden
- rejection from loved ones
- pain
- disability
- death

Of course, every circumstance is unique and influenced by many factors. Some of your fears may be valid and worthy of your current attention, while other fears either aren't currently relevant or, even if they are relevant, are consuming you more than they should be. If you are struggling with debilitating health anxiety, my guess is that at least some of your fears don't deserve the amount of attention they are getting.

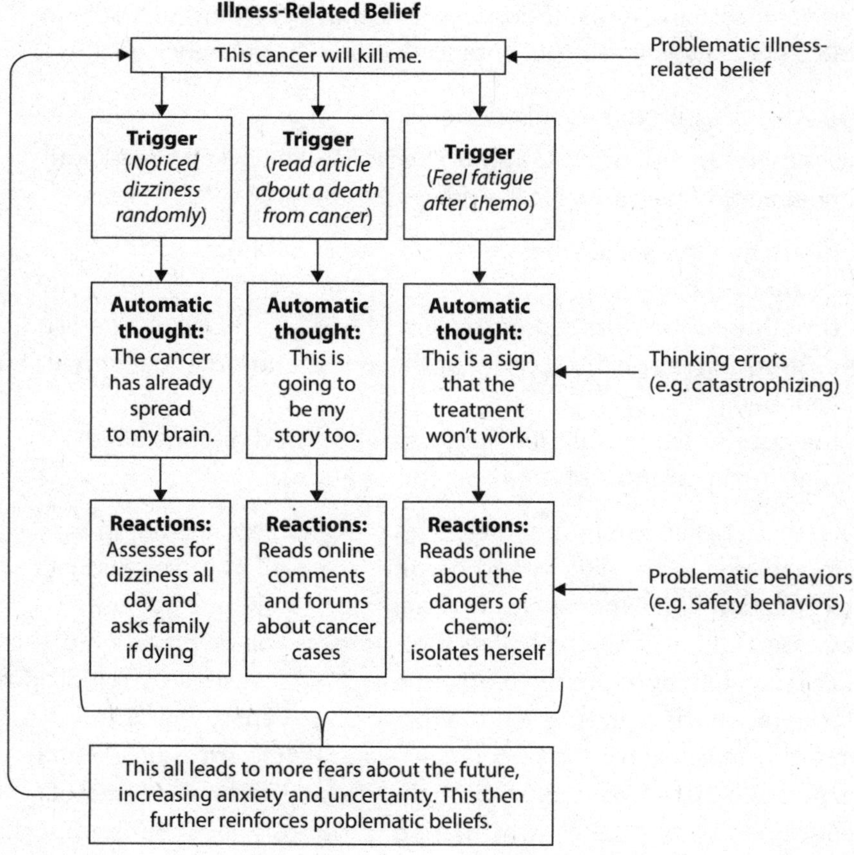
Illness-Related Belief
This cancer will kill me.
Problematic illness-related belief
Trigger (Noticed dizziness randomly)
Trigger (read article about a death from cancer)
Trigger (Feel fatigue after chemo)
Automatic thought: The cancer has already spread to my brain.
Automatic thought: This is going to be my story too.
Automatic thought: This is a sign that the treatment won't work.
Thinking errors (e.g. catastrophizing)
Reactions: Assesses for dizziness all day and asks family if dying
Reactions: Reads online comments and forums about cancer cases
Reactions: Reads online about the dangers of chemo; isolates herself
Problematic behaviors (e.g. safety behaviors)
This all leads to more fears about the future, increasing anxiety and uncertainty. This then further reinforces problematic beliefs.

By now, you know the cycle that takes place when we feel anxious about our health. This same cycle can be extremely problematic, even when we have a diagnosed medical condition. My client, Trang, had breast cancer. Despite a good prognosis and her diligence in following the treatment plan, she remained convinced that the cancer was going to kill her. This belief led her to be hypervigilant about her body, misinterpreting every new sensation or symptom as a sign that the cancer was spreading. As you can see in the diagram, getting stuck in this cycle consumed a lot of Trang's time and energy, ultimately deteriorating her emotional well-being and mental health.

It is more than understandable that Trang was anxious due to her cancer diagnosis and the treatment she had to endure. However, the anxiety had begun to chip away at her life and ultimately was having a negative impact on her physical and mental health. By dissecting and modifying certain beliefs, thoughts and behaviors, Trang was able to reduce her fears, increase her coping skills and improve her quality of life.

Constraining illness-related beliefs

The empirically supported Common Sense Model of Illness Self-Regulation[7] outlines a set of beliefs in five key areas:

1. **identity** or how the illness is labeled and its nature
2. **cause** of the illness
3. **timeline** or the duration of the illness (e.g. acute, chronic, episodic)
4. **consequences** or the severity of the illness and potential impact on well-being
5. the **cure** or extent that the illness can be cured or controlled (personally or through medical intervention).

Now, these beliefs are formed based on many factors, including the factors related to the disease and prognosis as well as the individual's interpretation and experiences. For example, if someone has been diagnosed with cancer, the beliefs they develop will be based on the very real circumstances of the cancer diagnosis as well as their own individual interpretations. However, given that people with anxiety tend to overestimate threat (or the hopelessness and helplessness of situations), it is possible that at least some of one's illness-related beliefs are not well-aligned with medical assessment or prognosis. If so, this is important to address, as illness-related beliefs help one make sense of their illness and guide coping strategies and reactions to circumstances throughout its course.[7]

Table 1 Examples of problematic illness-related beliefs

I deserve this disease.	There is nothing I can do to improve this disease.
I don't deserve to get better.	Treatment will not help me with this disease.
This disease is due to bad karma.	My life has no value anymore.
God/The Universe is punishing me with this disease.	I am no longer me/will never be me again.
I will never be able to cope with this symptom/this symptom will never end.	I will never be happy/fulfilled again.
I am bound to live in misery for the rest of my life.	This disease has made/will make me unlovable.
This disease will inevitably kill me.	This disease has made/will make me worthless.

Trang struggled with several constraining illness-related beliefs. We worked to change beliefs that were inaccurate and caused a lot of distress in her life. Of course, beliefs aren't always completely inaccurate. This is why it is helpful to evaluate them and modify them when it is necessary. If a distressing belief is true, then we work on taking actionable steps to improve the situation as well as coping.

Evaluating and challenging problematic thoughts

We interpret our day-to-day experiences with our health condition through the lens of our beliefs. As you know, problematic beliefs can lead us to engage in many different thinking errors, which in turn lead to maladaptive emotional and behavioral reactions. Below are a few examples of how thinking errors can play out while dealing with a medical condition.

Overgeneralization: fearing that a disease outcome you heard about in the media means that your outcome will be the same.

Catastrophizing: assuming the absolute worst possible disease outcome even without substantial evidence for it or when evidence suggests the contrary (e.g. your doctor's prognosis doesn't suggest the worst-case scenario). Or assuming the worst-case scenario when it comes to coping (e.g. you will live in misery for the rest of your life, you will never feel better).

Mental filter/Tunnel vision: focusing on situations in which treatment for the disease didn't work and paying less attention to the cases in which treatment was effective.

Jumping to conclusions: every bodily sensation or bodily change, even when minor or irrelevant, makes you think that the disease is progressing/returning.

Emotional reasoning: assuming that your feeling proves the state of your disease, the reason for symptoms or the success of treatment (e.g. something feels wrong, therefore these test results are going to be bad news).

Labeling: giving yourself unfair/inaccurate labels because you are facing this disease (e.g. this disease makes me helpless, worthless, unlovable).

Magical thinking: beliefs that thoughts/acts will influence unrelated events (e.g. I got this disease because of karma; if I am extra kind this month, my condition will improve).

All-or-nothing thinking: seeing yourself, the disease or symptoms as dichotomous instead of on a continuum (e.g. my body must be broken/useless or I wouldn't have this disease).

Disqualifying/discounting the positive: Dismissing the positives of a situation related to your health (e.g. my doctor said my labs look good but he was just trying to make me feel better).

Once you identify thinking errors, challenge them with Socratic dialogue, as we have been doing in most of the chapters throughout this book. Continue building the habit of critically analyzing your thoughts and looking for inconsistencies or inaccuracies and then make the necessary changes. Below are a few questions you can use to help you challenge any potentially distorted thoughts when it comes to your health condition. The goal is to find the most adaptive and helpful way of viewing a situation.

Table 2 Examples of Socratic questions to challenge thoughts related to health condition

- What is the evidence that this thought about my health is true? Is there any evidence against this thought?
- What is the effect of me having this thought (about a symptom, the disease, my future)? What could be the effect of me changing this thought?
- Am I hyper focusing on stories about people who were diagnosed with the same condition as me and had poor outcomes and not considering all of the others who received treatment and recovered or managed it well?
- What is the worst-case scenario for my medical condition, considering the disease, doctor's prognosis, treatment plan/progress? What is the best-case scenario? What is the most likely scenario?
- Does my assumption (about a symptom, my disease or me) represent black-and-white thinking (perfect health or serious illness)? Is there a more nuanced way of seeing this?
- Have I coped with challenges in the past? What strengths do I have that have helped me overcome adversity before? How can I apply these to coping with this health issue?
- How can I or have I been able to emotionally cope with this disease? What has helped me to cope with illness/struggles in the past?
- How can I or have I been able to physically cope with this disease? What medical resources will allow me to manage, treat and/or overcome this disease? What would it look like to cope and live well with my condition?

Distinguishing between health anxiety and valid health concerns

You might rationalize that having a medical diagnosis means it is necessary and perhaps even responsible to worry about or look into every bodily change. This is not true. Yes, you should be mindful of and responsive to certain types of symptoms, depending on your specific circumstances. However, every bodily sensation should not be considered a crisis. A person can have a medical condition and also have health anxiety that is excessive beyond the threat of the disease. In fact, medical conditions and severe health anxiety (i.e. somatic symptom disorder) are common comorbidities.[8,9]

To reduce anxiety about symptoms, it can help to have a conversation with your physician about valid concerns related to your diagnosis. During this conversation, ask your physician to clearly describe the symptoms that would warrant an emergency or office medical visit based on your medical condition. You can also tell your doctor about the types of symptoms/sensations or bodily changes that you worry signify an urgent concern related to your medical condition. Your doctor can then clarify and reduce anxiety over any unnecessary concerns about bodily sensations. Refer to the form in Chapter 8. Next time you meet with your doctor, bring the worksheet as a guide.

Having these conversations with your doctor can free you from the burden of assuming that every symptom, sensation or bodily change is a sign that your health condition has worsened. Symptoms or sensations outside of what your doctor has expressed concern about can be treated in the way we have discussed in earlier chapters. Specifically, consider the common sources of body noise discussed in Chapter 5. Further, consider the symptoms that call for immediate medical attention in Chapter 8. After consulting with your doctor, if you find yourself feeling anxious about a symptom that your doctor didn't express concerns about, ask yourself some of the questions in the table below.

Table 3 Questions to address health concerns

- What thoughts ran through my mind when I first noticed this symptom or these symptoms? Could these thoughts be intensifying the symptoms?
- After reviewing the list of symptoms associated with random bodily noise and/or anxiety or the fight-or-flight response in Chapter 5, is it possible that these bodily sensations could be due to benign bodily fluctuations and changes?
- What are my normal physiological responses to anxiety (i.e. my specific patterns)? Is it possible that my current bodily sensation or symptom is a part of my normal pattern of response to an anxiety trigger?
- Could there be other, harmless or benign explanations for these symptoms such as caffeine intake, change in diet, lack of sleep or stress?
- Did my doctor link any of these symptoms to my medical condition and something I should seek medical consultation for?
- Could this symptom be due to an minor illness or issue that is unrelated to my medical condition?

If you find yourself in the pattern of hyper focusing on a symptom that has been cleared by your doctor (i.e. is not one of the symptoms your doctor said is a concern or requires medical attention), then you can try the waiting experiment discussed in Chapter 7. Practice pausing and refraining from searching for answers for a select number of days. At the end of the waiting period, you can always schedule an appointment with your doctor if the symptom persists or you are concerned. This exercise will allow you to get out of the habit of assuming that every new sensation is related to your medical condition or needs to be immediately addressed.

Distinguishing between productive and unproductive worry

When you are dealing with a medical condition, you face a wide range of new stressors on top of your existing responsibilities. This can lead to a lot of new stress and worry. Sometimes this worry can be incredibly unproductive, particularly when we enter a downward spiral of worry thoughts about all kinds of potential worst-case scenarios and feel compelled to find solutions for all of these 'what ifs.' We talked about the unproductive worry cycle in Chapter 7. However, worry can be productive at times and, in these cases, it can prompt problem-solving and help one find solutions.

It can be helpful to evaluate our worry thoughts and distinguish between productive and unproductive worry. Below are a few key characteristics of each type of worry,[10,11,12] along with a couple of examples to illustrate.

Productive worry

- Worry regarding current, tangible problems
- Focus on issues we have some degree of influence over
- Aim to problem-solve and identify solutions
- Able to accept imperfect solutions
- Confidence in one's ability to handle challenges effectively
- Accompanied by low levels of stress and anxiety

Leticia is about to begin dialysis treatments several times per week. She is worried about the logistics of getting childcare for her kids during these appointments, as her spouse works. She also worries about how to make adjustments in her life to cover the additional medical bills. She and her spouse schedule a family meeting to discuss getting help from loved ones with watching children during her dialysis appointments. Leticia also makes an appointment with the social worker at the dialysis treatment center to explore options in terms of accessing financial assistance. Essentially, her worries are about immediate, tangible problems, which leads to problem-solving to identify potential solutions.

Unproductive worry

- Worry regarding distant, abstract scenarios
- Focus on problems we have little or no control over
- Reject solutions because can't be certain about outcome
- Heavy focus on the negative emotions around the worry situation
- Feel helpless and doubt our ability to cope
- Accompanied by high levels of stress and anxiety

Eric has Type 2 diabetes. He is young and has been responsibly managing his illness with lifestyle changes and medication. However, he often sinks into a cycle of worry about random, distant potential negative or catastrophic events related to his illness. He worries about something going wrong in the future with his body because of diabetes, such as a heart attack, stroke or kidney failure. He worries about whether in these future scenarios he won't be well enough to enjoy his retirement years or play with his future grandchildren. Despite his doctor's assurances that he is managing his disease well and, therefore, reducing risk of future comorbidities, his worries about these distant scenarios create overwhelming anxiety, making him feel helpless.

Let's do an exercise. Pick one or two of your worry thoughts that have come up recently about your health. Run them through this test. Based on these characteristics, which category did they fall into? Write them down and label them as productive or unproductive worry. For unproductive worry thoughts, search for any potential thinking errors and use the Socratic questions from earlier in this chapter to help you challenge these types of unhelpful worry thoughts. For productive worries, ask yourself a few questions:

- What can I control in this situation?
- What are the immediate/current problems that need to be addressed?
- Are there actionable steps I can take to address this/these problem(s)? Make a list of actionable steps I can take to begin identifying potential solutions.

'Twist and Finish out the Image' technique

When we catastrophize about our health, we often picture the worst-case scenario and then abruptly end the daydream at the worst point in the scenario. We talked about this in Chapter 5 when we introduced this technique. Dealing with health anxiety and a real medical condition can even further exacerbate this tendency and lead us to imagine all sorts of worst-case scenarios related to our diagnosis. We want to redirect the impulse to automatically conjure up worst-case scenario imagery and, instead, build a habit of imagining a more realistic and positive conclusion to daydreams about future scenarios with our health.

Rudy, a client of mine with health anxiety who had recently been diagnosed with cancer, would sometimes slip into a habit of imagining the worst-case scenario. In these moments when his anxiety was high, he would skip everything in between and go through an abbreviated, two-step process: 1) gets diagnosed with cancer; and 2) dies from cancer. And that was that. However, there were so many more variations of his situation that were not only plausible but more likely, given his prognosis and treatment options.

To address this tendency, Rudy finished out the image of getting treatment for cancer and added a positive, more realistic twist to the story. He imagined himself going through treatment several times per week. He imagined all the love and support he would receive from his family during this very challenging time. He imagined himself getting his last round of chemo and how he went to dinner with his wife to celebrate afterward. Lastly, he imagined himself walking into his oncologist's office, who informed him that the scans indicated that treatment was effective and he was now in remission. He imagined his wife squeezing his hand and smiling as they received the good news. As they drove home, he imagined himself having a whole new sense of gratitude for his life, given everything he had been through.

When it comes to your fears about your own diagnosis, how do you catastrophize? What is your abbreviated process? Think of a situation recently in which you had catastrophic thoughts about your diagnosis, ending the daydream at the worst point in the scenario. Perhaps you were in misery while managing the disease, died or were in the dying process. Write out the scenario. Next, you will twist the story as necessary and finish it out on a more realistic and/or positive note. Remember, this technique will be difficult at first. It takes time to reshape thinking, but the more you learn to think in this way, the easier it will get over time.

Table 3 Twist and Finish Out the Image

Situation/trigger	What happened and how did it end?	How can you twist the narrative and finish out the story?

Dialing down catastrophic thinking

When we catastrophize, we overestimate just how awful the outcome will be. However, we cannot let catastrophic thoughts run wild in our mind, as they will take over and make us miserable. What's more, by not intervening in this thought process, you are allowing your brain to develop and maintain a terrible habit. The more power you give to these types of thoughts, the more these thinking patterns get solidified and, thus, the easier it becomes for your brain to catastrophize in the future.

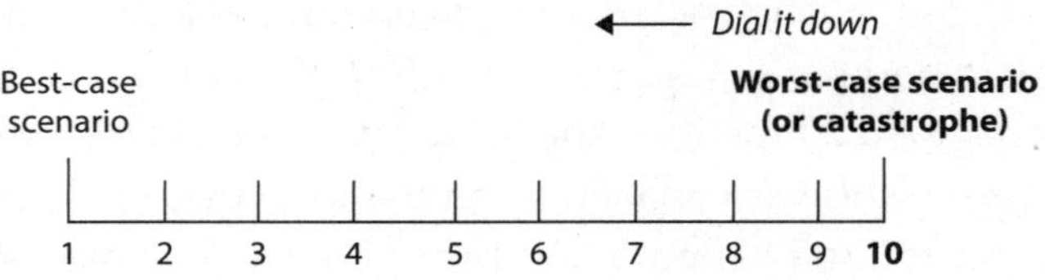

Let's try dialing down the catastrophic thinking. Sometimes an image can help illustrate a concept. We will oversimplify this idea by using a scale. Think of your thoughts as being on a scale from 1–10 in terms of the outcome you are picturing. Think of '1' as the best-case scenario. Think of '10' as the worst-case scenario (i.e. your catastrophic thought). In this exercise, you don't need to dial it all the way down to a '1' or the absolute best-case scenario. Simply dial it down a bit, perhaps to a 7 or a 6, just a few notches.

As you'll see in the examples below, you don't need to arrive at the best-case scenario. Remember, changing thinking patterns isn't about positive thinking but more realistic thinking. The 'dialed down' thought should simply be the more realistic outcome. The next time you have a catastrophic thought, try dialing it down to an outcome that is less extreme.

Table 4 Managing thoughts

Catastrophic thought	Dialed-down thought
Getting sick is a sign that my disease is progressing.	Getting sick is a normal part of life, whether someone has a medical condition or not.
If I don't recover quickly from this procedure, it means I will be disabled for the rest of my life.	Even if I don't recover quickly within the typical timeframe, I will still likely be in a better position than I am now.
This disease is going to kill me.	Given all my treatment options, I will most likely live.
This chemo is killing me.	This chemo has side effects and is weakening my immune system.
This pain will never go away.	I have good days and bad days. It will probably continue that way.

Gratitude journaling

I once heard someone say, '*People with anxiety do their best when they stay as close to the present moment as possible.*' This resonated with me, and I never forgot it. Why is it important to stay in the present moment? Well, anxiety tends to be future-oriented.

With health anxiety, in particular, we fear disease, whether we have one or not, ultimately because we fear the disease will either make us or our loved ones miserable and/or will lead to death. Regardless of the reason we do it, spending the majority of the time in the future is not adaptive or helpful. In the mental health sphere, we place a lot of emphasis on mindfulness and present-centeredness. This is because we only have 'right now.' The more time we are able to focus on the present moment, the less we will focus on all the future 'what ifs.' Learning to do this takes practice.

One helpful daily exercise that can help you practice living in the moment is gratitude journaling. I recommend doing this daily for a couple of weeks to develop the habit. Pick a time of day to do this routine. Some of my clients prefer to do it in the morning as a refreshing way to start their day. Other clients like to do it in the evening as a way to reflect on their day and get into the right mindset before bed. In a journal (or on piece of paper or notepad on your phone), list 3–5 things you are grateful for right now. It might be, 'I like the sound of my kids stomping around upstairs' or 'I like the flavor of this new coffee creamer.' Keep it simple and easy so that you will continue doing it. The more consistent you are with this, the more you will get used to a present-focused thinking habit.

Reshaping illness-related beliefs

We discussed earlier how constraining illness-related beliefs can have a detrimental impact on our daily lives. We must continue to use techniques to improve the daily, surface-level automatic thoughts and behaviors. However, we must also target deeper-level cognitions about the disease we have, the underlying illness-related beliefs. In this section, we will provide an example of how to use the core belief worksheet to modify an illness-related belief, but for detailed instructions on how to use this technique, refer to Chapter 3.

My client, Ainsley, struggled with fibromyalgia and dealt with a lot of pain. She had good days and bad days. On her bad days, she would sometimes have to miss work and social activities with her friends and family. She had anxiety about this, as she worried that her husband and other loved ones were going to get tired of her being sick and unable to do things. We did some digging and realized that one of Ainsley's illness-related beliefs was that fibromyalgia was changing her, making her unlovable and unworthy. We decided to unpack and reconsider this belief with a core belief worksheet.

Old core belief

THIS DISEASE IS MAKING ME UNLOVABLE AND UNWORTHY.

How much do you believe this core belief (*before the intervention*)? (0–100) **70**

EVIDENCE THAT SEEMS TO SUPPORT THE OLD CORE BELIEF (WITH REFRAME)

- There are many things I used to do that made me who I am (e.g. going to shows, playing guitar, singing, biking, swimming, hosting parties and events). I still do the same things but not as often as I used to. When I am in pain or experiencing fatigue, I am not the same energetic person I used to be. *REFRAME: I am still me even when I don't feel like me. There have been many times before I had these symptoms and this diagnosis that I didn't feel like myself. For example, I didn't feel like myself when I was having a bad week, did badly on a test, lost a job or got dumped. I wasn't any less 'me' then. I was just me but more tired or grumpy, lol. In the same way, I am still me even when I am tired or not feeling well.*

- At times, I don't feel like myself in social situations. I am usually the outgoing one in the group and lately I just am more on the quiet side. I also usually love to laugh and I just don't find things as funny lately. I worry that the 'me' as I know it is fading out. *REFRAME: Like the point above, this is emotional reasoning—confusing feelings with facts. Not feeling like myself doesn't make me any less 'me.' I am still who I am no matter what mood I am in or what situation I am in. I am allowed to have bad days just like everyone else. No one is their best self all the time.*
- My family, friends and husband may get tired of dealing with the 'sick' person. If the symptoms and challenges of the disease worsen, they could reject me. *REFRAME: People that truly love us don't abandon us because we go through something hard. It may be tiring or difficult at times to support me with ongoing challenges and that is okay. It doesn't mean they will abandon me. I can also remind myself that if the tables were turned, I would support any of my loved ones (and have)... even if it is hard sometimes.*

How much do you believe this core belief (*after the intervention*)? (0–100) 45

New core belief

THIS DISEASE DOESN'T CHANGE WHO I AM—VALUABLE AND WORTHY OF LOVE.

How much do you believe this core belief (*before the intervention*)? (0–100) 15

EVIDENCE THAT CONTRADICTS THE OLD CORE BELIEF AND SUPPORTS THE NEW ONE

- I am a valuable, worthy, lovable and capable human being, regardless of how I interpret things or how I feel in the moment.

All human beings have the same value. My circumstances, struggles, thoughts, beliefs and feelings don't determine my value. My value stays the same. The only thing that changes is whether I am able to see my value clearly enough or not.

- Even though on some days (when I have more pain) it has been difficult to feel like myself, on other days I am still able to be 'me' in many ways. I still make my dumb and sometimes funny jokes and am social with people. Even my colleague commented on it when I was leaving work early—she said, wow,' I didn't know you weren't feeling well.' I still am who I am, whether sick or not. I just forget that sometimes.
- There are other days in which I don't feel sick at all. On those days, I feel like my usual self and it feels really good.
- My loved ones have already shown me (currently and in the past) that they won't abandon me when times get hard. They've been there for me in dealing with these health challenges. They were also there for me through many challenges I've had to face in the past. They have never made me feel disposable. And I have treated them the same way. I have healthy relationships and we support each other. But, importantly, even if someone close to me did see me as not valuable or not worthy of love because of my health challenges, that would say more about them than me. Someone else's actions do not determine my value.
- When my husband got into a car accident, he sustained many injuries and wasn't able to work or do a lot of the same activities for almost six months. Although it was hard, this did not change my love for him or my commitment to our relationship. I need to remember that when I worry about being an inconvenience.

How much do you believe this core belief (*after the intervention*)? (0–100) **75**

Waiting for test results

Waiting for test results can be awful for anyone with health anxiety. It can be especially stressful when you are managing a medical condition. It is understandable that you would fear receiving bad news related to your condition. Of course, waiting for test results puts you in an anxiety-provoking situation, which inevitably makes you more vulnerable to problematic thinking and behavior.

You might start to catastrophize, envisioning all sorts of worst-case scenarios, or engage in excessive worry in which you try to anticipate and plan for every possible outcome. You also might engage in unhelpful behaviors, like incessantly checking the online portal or your phone as you wait for the results. Or perhaps you find yourself excessively checking your body or reading all about your disease. Contrarily, you might take the opposite approach and avoid getting the results or engage in unhelpful behaviors such as numbing your mind with alcohol or drugs to avoid thinking about it. Any of this can make you utterly miserable.

Challenging thoughts and limiting behaviors

It may come as no shock to you that I want you to, first and foremost, pay attention to the thoughts and behaviors that are popping up while waiting for your test results. It can be helpful to start with the feeling. If you are feeling overwhelming anxiety during this waiting period, ask yourself: what was just going through my mind? Identify the automatic thought and then look through the list of thinking errors at

Table 5 Managing anxiety over test results

- What is the evidence that my prediction about the test results is true? Is there any evidence against this thought?
- Is there another way to view the situation?
- What is the effect of me having this thought about the test results? What could be the effect of me changing this thought?
- Am I selectively remembering the stories about people who were given bad news about their test results? Am I considering all the people who received neutral or good news?
- Am I assuming that my feelings right now are predicting the results of the test? How often have my feelings been wrong in the past?
- Am I thinking of test results in a black-or-white way (e.g. amazing/perfect results or complete catastrophe)? Is there a more nuanced way of seeing this?
- Am I only focused on the worst-case scenario for my test results? What is the best-case scenario? What is the most likely/realistic scenario?
- What are my most effective coping strategies (that are also healthy) that I can use while waiting for these test results? My social support system, personal resilience, faith, therapy, support groups, self-help books, personal hobbies, treats?

the beginning of this chapter. Are any relevant? Write them down. Next, challenge them.

In addition to identifying and challenging thoughts, pay attention to what you *do* when you start to feel anxious about the test results. Are you searching for studies on the internet, asking loved ones what they think, engaging in body vigilance to look for signs or indications that your test results won't be good? As you know, these behaviors seem like they might help you but will only make your anxiety worse. Try to refrain from them and refer to the techniques in Chapter 6 for help if you need it.

Examples of how to reframe thoughts related to testing:

1 I've been feeling off lately, so that must mean the test results will be bad. *REFRAME: Many things can cause symptoms and they don't necessarily mean something serious. I will wait for the results before jumping to conclusions or assuming my emotions are predictive of outcomes.*
2 If the test results are bad, my life is over. *REFRAME: Even if the results are not what I hope, there are treatments and ways to manage. Many people face health challenges and continue to live meaningful lives. It is not all bad or all good.*
3 If the results are bad, I won't be able to handle it. *REFRAME: I've handled difficult situations before and found ways to cope. No matter the result, I have the strength to deal with it, and I have support.*
4 Waiting is unbearable. I can't think about anything else until I know the results. *REFRAME: Waiting is uncomfortable, but it's temporary. I can focus on other areas of my life, healthy distractions and self-care during this time to reduce anxiety. Worrying won't make the results come any faster.*
5 This test is everything. My entire future depends on it. *REFRAME: This test is important, but it's one piece of the puzzle. Whatever the outcome, there are next steps and options available.*

Compartmentalizing and present-centeredness

If you find yourself stuck in a cycle of problematic thoughts and behaviors while waiting for test results, you can compartmentalize. Compartmentalizing is a defense mechanism used to reduce anxiety by placing unpleasant thoughts or emotions into 'boxes' to be opened up at another time. You might hear some experts caution against this strategy. Indeed, it can become an unhealthy coping method, particularly when you use it as a long-term solution to avoid any negative emotions or thoughts, leading to unaddressed problems.

However, it can be used as an effective tool to manage stress and anxiety. After all, there are times in which it would be unhelpful to face and unpack heavy emotions and distressing thoughts. For example, if you are going through a divorce, it can be beneficial to set those feelings aside while you are finishing an important task at work.

You can compartmentalize while waiting for your test results by choosing to (temporarily) put 'thinking about the results' into the 'box' and placing it on the proverbial shelf. The reason this can be helpful is because there is nothing you can do at this time to influence the results of the test. Ruminating on it has zero influence on the outcome and merely causes distress. Use that energy and time to do something else instead, something that keeps you present-focused. Is there a hobby or favorite activity you can spend time doing? Is there a friend you thoroughly enjoy spending time with who can help keep you focused on the present moment? Is there a movie you have been waiting to see? Is there some way you can treat yourself? One of my clients decided to go with a good friend to an amusement park and ride roller coasters all day.

Addressing problematic behaviors

When you have a medical condition, it can be very easy to rationalize safety behaviors and avoidance even though they foster dependence, reinforce dysfunctional beliefs and ultimately create a vicious cycle. After all, a symptom *could* be a sign that your disease is progressing or returning. It therefore makes sense that you would excessively seek information, check your body and seek reassurance from others. Right? The problem with this rationale is that your body is still a human body that makes noise for random, benign or minor reasons. Yes, you have a disease that produces symptoms. But your human body also produces sensations and symptoms for a multitude of other reasons that have nothing to do with your disease.

This is why it can be helpful to have a conversation with your doctor(s) about the symptoms that constitute a concern when it comes to your health condition. I highly encourage you to do the exercise from earlier if you haven't yet. This can take the pressure off of you to assess every bodily sensation and decide whether you are safe or in danger. Once you know the specific symptoms or bodily changes to be aware of, you can free yourself from going down the rabbit hole for every sensation. We would want you to then approach symptoms in the same way we would want anyone to, whether they have a diagnosis or not. Use the techniques you learned in Chapter 6 to help you refrain from using safety behaviors.

Avoidance can be another common problem for people with medical conditions who also have health anxiety. The anxiety can make you avoid going to the doctor, getting testing done and participating in treatments. You might fear being told terrible news or experiencing discomfort, pain or anxiety during the testing or treatment process. Usually, the avoidance habit builds slowly. If you are like most cases, you didn't just wake up one day and say, 'I am never going to the doctor again.' You simply continue to put it off, which then makes the appointments grow scarier and more anxiety-producing over time. To overcome avoidance, gradually face your fear by taking it one baby step at a time. Use the guide in Chapter 8 to approach this with an exposure hierarchy.

Managing anxiety while getting testing and treatment

Getting diagnosed and treated for a life-altering or life-limiting diagnosis can be traumatic, having a negative impact on the way a person views and interacts with the medical setting. As we discussed in Chapter 8, medical trauma is uniquely challenging. It often requires that people remain in regular contact with the setting in which the trauma took place, particularly if you have a medical condition that requires you to get regular intervention. Perhaps you faced frightening and challenging experiences throughout the diagnostic or treatment process. It is understandable if these experiences have heightened your anxiety and made you fearful or hesitant to return to the medical setting.

If you leave these challenges unaddressed, you may avoid the medical system or interact with it in a problematic way and make yourself miserable. We want you to have some helpful tools to cope with any distress you might experience while getting testing and treatment. It can be beneficial to help you better understand your experiences while in the medical setting as well as help you develop coping skills and build a sense of empowerment. Getting you to a place in which you feel even a little bit safer and more empowered is a great goal.

Paying attention to triggers and thoughts

In Chapter 8, we discussed stimuli in medical settings that can trigger anxiety. If you've had scary and/or traumatic experiences, you may find that certain smells, sights or sounds are triggering. It can be helpful to explore this to gain an understanding of how these triggers impact you. This will help you cope with the impact of these triggers when you do face them, whether you expect them or are surprised by them. Hopefully the exercise in Chapter 8 gave you some insight into your own triggers and thoughts or thinking errors when you interact with the medical setting. It might be helpful to take a picture of your thought record and document your experiences of this when you go in for testing or treatment related to your diagnosis. This can help you challenge and reframe distressing thoughts and reduce your anxiety.

Contextualizing

Your experiences related to your diagnosis may have made you feel vulnerable. It can be especially difficult to re-enter the medical setting, particularly if it is the same setting in which you have endured scary or negative experiences. It is possible to be decontextualized while receiving intervention in the medical setting.[12] This means that you may feel powerless and unsafe because you are outside of your usual contexts in which you have some sense of control, familiarity or comfort. As a result, you might feel disconnected from the things that make you feel like *you*. To address this, it can be helpful to remain contextualized and reconnect with yourself while interacting with the medical setting.

Think through some of the things that are not only comforting but bring back a sense of who you are. The simple act of reconnecting with some of the things that emphasize *you* can be both empowering and create a sense of safety. As you look through the ideas below, make a list of whatever comes to mind. Then think through what would be feasible to bring to your medical appointments. Of course, this will vary depending on the type, duration and nature of your medical appointments.

Next, plan to pack a little 'comfort bag.' This bag might include physical items as well as digital items plus a list of all the digital/physical items you have included. You will bring this bag with you to your appointments. The goal is to have it bring some comfort as well as to serve as a reminder of who you are and where you come from.

As an example, one of my clients brought several comforting/familiar items to her chemotherapy appointments: her favorite *Friends* episode (downloaded on Netflix just in case the wi-fi was slow); a playlist of her favorite upbeat songs; a faith-based devotional book; a pumpkin spice candle; and a framed photo of a surprise party all her friends threw for her when she got her graduate degree. These items helped get her through the first few appointments, which she was very anxious about.

Table 6 Ideas for the comfort bag

Your favorites	What are your favorite snacks, drinks, colors, seasons, animals, books, TV shows, music, movies, actors, authors, quotes? You could bring various favorite items, whether in physical or digital form.
People you love	Who are the people in your life that bring you the most comfort? You could bring someone to your appointment, bring pictures, videos or other reminders of them (their scent, a piece of clothing, a fond memory you have together, a video/audio message/text from them that you love (or they could create it specially for you to get through that day)).
Comforting scents	Are there scents that bring you comfort—your perfume/cologne or a loved one's perfume/cologne, a type of laundry soap, body spray, candle, shampoo/conditioner, lotion, food/drink?
Items from home	Are there comforting items from home—a blanket, a special mug, slippers, a candle, a stuffed animal, small flower or plant?
Activities/ Entertainment	Are there certain activities you love to engage in that you could bring—crossword puzzles, TV shows, movies, songs or playlists, podcasts, YouTube channels, fiction books, board games?

Faith/Spirituality	Is there anything connected to your faith or spirituality that brings comfort—scripture, prayers, inspiring messages, books, videos, podcasts, workbooks, rituals, music?
Food/Drinks	Are there food/drinks that bring pleasure and/or comfort—snacks, treats, specialty coffee or tea?
Memories	What are your favorite memories? Think of good times with your family, spouse, friends; or from college, vacations, holidays, celebratory events, intimate moments; memories that were hilarious, moments of growth, bonding with others, proud moments, challenges that paid off, something special someone said to you. You could bring items that represent these memories—pictures/albums, keepsakes, souvenirs, letters, art, videos.

Patient advocacy

Navigating healthcare systems can be complicated, disorienting and frustrating. The process of dealing with insurance companies, new financial burdens and/or the logistics of medical testing, diagnosis and/or treatment are especially overwhelming while in the middle of trying to psychologically and physically cope with a medical condition. It can be helpful to have an advocate help you handle these challenges, if possible.

In the USA, a patient advocate (or patient navigator) can help guide you through the healthcare system during screening, diagnosis, treatment and follow-up. They might assist with communicating with healthcare providers (e.g. gather info and ask the right questions to guide your decision-making, speak up for you) or introduce you to psychological and social support as well as medical, financial and legal resources. They can also help by working with insurance companies, case managers, social workers, lawyers, employers and other relevant people involved. See the appendix for resources to get connected with a patient advocate.

In addition to finding your own advocate based on your condition or as a part of the patient advocate foundation or an outside advocacy group, many healthcare facilities have patient advocates on staff in addition to social workers, nurse case managers and an internal ombudsman that can assist with accessing resources and understanding complex systems. Loved ones can also act as an ally by educating themselves, attending medical appointments with you, asking direct questions and taking notes as well as serving as a chief coordinator for all medical, financial and legal matters. Lastly, if you have a therapist or want to begin therapy, they can also advocate for you. For example, a therapist may write a letter to your provider making a special request during treatment as necessary (e.g. presence of family members, technology or comfort items).

Therapy and support groups

Therapy can be a helpful resource after receiving a life-altering or life-limiting diagnosis or while navigating medical systems. Your therapist can help you build essential skills to manage your anxiety and overwhelm during this challenging time in your life. They can help you process and cope with the changes you are going through. Your therapist can also help you in your relationships with loved ones as necessary. For example, therapists will often invite a partner or another family member to join in on a session to help improve communication and find solutions to problems in the relationship. Lastly, group therapy or support groups are a way to connect with others who are going through a similar struggle. Hospitals and other healthcare facilities often have clinical social workers, therapists and group facilitators on staff. See the appendix for resources on finding a therapist or group.

References

1 Hughes L, Taylor RM, Beckett AE, Lindner OC, Martin A, McCulloch J, Morgan S, Soanes L, Uddin R, Stark DP. The Emotional Impact of a Cancer Diagnosis: A Qualitative Study of Adolescent and Young Adult Experience. Cancers (Basel). 2024 Mar 29;16(7):1332. doi: 10.3390/cancers16071332. PMID: 38611010; PMCID: PMC11010824.

2 Riba, M. B., Donovan, K. A., Ahmed, K., Andersen, B., Braun, II., Breitbart, W. S., Brewer, B. W., Corbett, C., Fann, J., Fleishman, S., Garcia, S., Greenberg, D. B., Handzo, G. F., Hoofring, L. H., Huang, C. H., Hutchinson, S., Johns, S., Keller, J., Kumar, P., ... Darlow, S. D. (2023). NCCN GUIDELINES® INSIGHTS Distress Management, Version 2.2023. *JNCCN Journal of the National Comprehensive Cancer Network, 21*(5), 450–457. https://doi.org/10.6004/jnccn.2023.0026

3 Martin R, Rothrock NE, Leventhal H, Leventhal EA. Common Sense Models of Illness: Implications for Symptom Perception and Health-Related

Behaviors. *Blackwell Publishing Ltd eBooks*. Published online December 24, 2009:199–225. doi:https://doi.org/10.1002/9780470753552.ch8

4 Baines T, Wittkowski A. A Systematic Review of the Literature Exploring Illness Perceptions in Mental Health Utilising the Self-Regulation Model. *Journal of Clinical Psychology in Medical Settings*. 2012;20(3):263–274. doi:https://doi.org/10.1007/s10880-012-9337-9

5 Wright LM, Bell JM: Beliefs and illness : a model for healing. [Calgary]: 4th Floor Press; 2009.

6 Järemo P, Arman M, Gerdle B, Larsson B, Gottberg K. Illness beliefs among patients with chronic widespread pain - associations with self-reported health status, anxiety and depressive symptoms and impact of pain. *BMC Psychology*. 2017;5. doi:https://doi.org/10.1186/s40359-017-0192-1

7 Hagger MS, Koch S, Chatzisarantis NLD, Orbell S. The common sense model of self-regulation: Meta-analysis and test of a process model. *Psychological Bulletin*. 2017;143(11):1117–1154. doi:https://doi.org/10.1037/bul0000118

8 Pandey S, Parikh MN, Brahmbhatt MJ, Vankar GK. Clinical study of illness anxiety disorder in medical outpatients. Archives of Psychiatry and Psychotherapy. 2017;19(4):32–41. doi:10.12740/APP/76932.

9 Lebel S, Mutsaers B, Tomei C, et al. Health anxiety and illness-related fears across diverse chronic illnesses: A systematic review on conceptualization, measurement, prevalence, course, and correlates. Kavushansky A, ed. *PLOS ONE*. 2020;15(7). doi:https://doi.org/10.1371/journal.pone.0234124

10 Davey GCL, Hampton J, Farrell J, Davidson S. Some characteristics of worrying: Evidence for worrying and anxiety as separate constructs. *Personality and Individual Differences*. 1992;13(2):133–147. doi:https://doi.org/10.1016/0191-8869(92)90036-o'

11 Clark DA, Beck AT. *Cognitive Therapy of Anxiety Disorders: Science and Practice*. Guilford Press; 2010.

12 Hall, MF, Hall, SE. Managing the Psychological Impact of Medical Trauma: A Guide for Mental Health and Healthcare Professionals. Springer Publishing; 2020.

Conclusion

You should be very proud of yourself for finishing this book. We covered a lot and I am sure some of these exercises were not easy to complete. My hope is that the concepts and skills you learned have helped improve your health anxiety. I specifically hope you have learned to see health and illness in fresh, new, healthier ways as well as learned how to replace problematic behaviors with those that are more helpful and adaptive.

Some of the key lessons I hope you will take away from this book:

- Serious disease is not as likely or severe as we often assume.
- Bodies make 'noise' for benign or minor reasons and sensations, most of which are not indicative of a medical crisis or underlying disease.
- Attaining certainty about symptoms or our health status is not possible, nor is it necessary to be safe.
- Coping behaviors like excessive body checking, reassurance-seeking and medical catastrophe prevention aren't necessary to keep us safe and they increase our anxiety over time.
- Death is a normal part of life and learning to accept it and to trust in our ability to cope with it when it happens can reduce health anxiety.
- It is necessary to build a reasonable amount of trust in healthcare and/or the ability of medical resources to help us cope with disease.
- Although medical conditions can be especially challenging to face, they are not synonymous with debilitating anxiety, misery and/or death.

Maintaining progress

It can sometimes be hard to see the bigger picture and recognize the progress we have made over time. It might help to take a few moments to think about the extent of your health anxiety when you started this book versus now. Were there any concepts in this book that were particularly helpful? Are there any skills you developed that have been especially useful in managing your anxiety? What aspects of your health anxiety still need more work?

Take note of any progress you have made. Give yourself credit. Write down what has changed. It is important to celebrate all of the small wins along your health anxiety journey. In fact, it is the accumulation of all the small wins that makes up your total progress over time. Don't dismiss the little changes you make in your day-to-day life. As you might have heard me say before, we improve anxiety by making small changes in our thoughts and behaviors every day. Another reason it is important to pay attention to your successes is we want to know what is working for you. Everyone is different. Some of the strategies in this book may have really resonated with you while others weren't as helpful. Knowing what works for you will help you to focus on those strategies going forward.

Once you recognize any progress you have made and what strategies worked best, you can continue the good work. You must exercise and refine your new skills. As with any new skill, the more you practice, the better you will get at it. It is essential that you work on these skills a little every day, week, month. If you don't, the concepts and skills learned in this book will simply fade into a distant, faint memory like most things do. The good news is that the more you practice these skills, the more you will retrain your brain and solidify long-term changes in your thinking and behavioral patterns. Over time and with practice, adaptive thinking and behavior will require less effort and become more of a natural response.

I encourage you to enlist the support of your loved ones as you continue on your journey to recovery. It is important to ask for help, although I know it isn't always easy. Having a support system can provide encouragement, inspiration and keep you from feeling alone and isolating yourself. People struggling with addiction need social support to help them from relapsing. This is just as valuable for those dealing with other mental health issues. It can also be helpful for loved ones to have an accurate understanding of what is happening 'behind the scenes' of health anxiety so they don't inadvertently feed your anxiety, such as by offering reassurance or encouraging unhelpful thoughts and behaviors. This is especially important for partners who likely interact with you the most (see helpful tips for partners in the appendix).

Improving your quality of life

Improving anxiety does not guarantee that one is living a happy or fulfilling life. Of course, the main goal of this book is to help you reduce your health anxiety so that it does not impair your ability to function 'normally' or sufficiently. However, even if you have succeeded in reducing anxiety about your health, you might have grown accustomed to a life that is deficient in joy, satisfaction and/or personal fulfillment. When we are highly anxious, we spend a lot of our time in 'survival mode.' This can make it difficult to prioritize the things that make us feel more alive, so to speak.

On a more basic level, one way to improve your sense of well-being is to ensure that you are taking a balanced approach when it comes to your physical and mental health, as we discussed in Chapter 6. This involves engaging in regular physical activity, eating a balanced and nutritious diet, getting enough sleep and refraining from drugs and excess alcohol use, and following all the recommendations to manage your physical health, such as getting screenings, check-ups and requirements to manage any existing health conditions.

Examples of taking a balanced approach to optimize your mental health are engaging in activities that make you feel fulfilled and/or build confidence, being intentional about staying connected with loved ones to the extent that it fits your personality and bandwidth, living a life that is aligned with your personal values and priorities as well as getting additional social support as is necessary through therapy, support groups, spirituality and/or faith-based activities.

It is worth emphasizing that enjoyable activities are an essential part of your overall quality of life. It is easy for many of us to disregard the important role this plays but clinical anxiety makes it particularly difficult to prioritize these activities. It can be helpful to reflect on the presence of 'positive activities' in your life. What types of activities bring you the most pleasure or excite you? How much of your daily/weekly/monthly life is filled with these types of activities? If you were to list out and reflect on your activities for each waking hour over the past week, is there anything you are doing too much or too little of?

Consider whether and to what extent you live a life of balance that optimizes your physical and mental health. Also, reflect on the extent to which you are satisfied and fulfilled. Can you make changes that would improve life satisfaction and overall well-being? Living a balanced life and giving yourself opportunities to be more fulfilled will help you maintain the progress you have made with health anxiety. Yes, some of these recommendations are obvious. But, as I always say to my clients, they are obvious for a reason.

Preparing for challenges and setbacks

Progress is not typically a linear process. You might be doing well with managing your health anxiety and then you face a new challenge or are triggered in some way, sending you stumbling backwards. This is normal and should be expected. I don't want you to be discouraged or feel hopeless if you feel more anxious about your health again at some point. Even with all the progress I have made over the years with my health anxiety, believe me, I still have my moments. But when this happens, I pull out the strategies from my little toolbox and get to work. My tools help me stop myself from spiraling.

Expect that setbacks are going to occur at various points in your life. You might be confronted with a new trigger, such as facing a health scare or getting diagnosed with a medical condition. Whatever the reason, I recommend you refer back to the strategies in this book when this happens. Try to see challenging moments as opportunities to use your adaptive coping strategies and refine your skills. Like I said in the beginning of this book, my goal is for you to develop a strong enough skill set to be your own CBT therapist. We don't want a setback propelling you back into a vicious cycle of dysfunctional thinking and behavior.

Accessing additional support

If you are still experiencing severe health anxiety after finishing this book, that is okay. I don't want you to get down on yourself about it, nor do I want you to lose hope in the prospect of getting better. Try to give yourself compassion. It took time and ongoing reinforcement to develop your thinking and behavioral patterns and, similarly, it may take some time and intentional effort to learn new patterns. That said, you may want to consider additional support to help you make progress on your health anxiety journey.

If you have the resources to do so, I would recommend connecting with a skilled CBT therapist who has expertise in treating health anxiety specifically. As discussed in the first chapter, CBT, including exposure therapy, is considered the first-line treatment for health anxiety. CBT can be delivered in either group or individual format, online or in-person and typically lasts between 10 and 20 sessions. Additional efficacious psychological treatments for health anxiety include stress management, mindfulness training, and acceptance and commitment therapy and can be offered online or in-person as well as in a group or individual format.[1]

Another option is to get a medication evaluation from a psychiatrist or other qualified healthcare professional. Certain pharmacological drugs have been shown to be effective in treating Illness Anxiety Disorder and are often used in combination with therapy.[2] Lastly, support groups are a way to connect with others who are also struggling with health anxiety, offering a sense of belonging and understanding. In the appendix you will find a list of resources for therapy, medication and support groups.

References

1 Tyrer P. Recent advances in the understanding and treatment of health anxiety. *Current Psychiatry Reports*. 2018;20(7). <https://doi.org/10.1007/s11920-018-0912-0>

2 French JH, Hameed S. Illness Anxiety Disorder. PubMed. Published 2020. <https://www.ncbi.nlm.nih.gov/books/NBK554399/>

Appendix

Tips for Loved Ones of People with Health Anxiety

People with health anxiety are, indeed, aware of how their anxiety impacts you, their loved one. It's not only exhausting for them but can be quite taxing on you as well. I remember my husband looking so fatigued at times because, for example, we had just spent half the afternoon talking about my health concerns. He hated to see me suffer and wanted to help but wasn't quite sure how. Also, on many of the occasions he was trying to help, he was inadvertently doing things that were counterproductive. He'd spend a lot of time trying to reassure me that I was okay, which (unbeknownst to him) was only making my anxiety worse. To add to all of that, loving someone with health anxiety can certainly be exhausting and frustrating at times. It can be hard not to get angry and lose patience. To help you support your loved one on their health anxiety journey, I will briefly outline a few unhelpful and helpful responses.

Unhelpful Responses or "Don'ts"

(1) Refrain from providing a lot of reassurance for symptoms

Of course, you are only doing this to help. However, reassurance-seeking is what is known as a "safety-seeking behavior." People with health anxiety use safety behaviors to reduce anxiety but ultimately these behaviors increase health anxiety. The health-anxious person becomes dependent on them and it ultimately just reinforces problematic beliefs. For example, by asking you 10 times in one week about whether you think a symptom is concerning, they unknowingly reinforce the idea that their health is constantly in danger and the only way to be "safe" is to seek reassurance from you or others.

Instead, we want them to learn how to reassure themself. We want them to use their own logic to challenge thoughts that they have a disease or are dying. This helps them learn to think in new ways. So, next time they ask you about a symptom, you can redirect the conversation. Ask them questions like: (1) "Well, what did your doctor say?" or (2) "How can you challenge this thought/worry of yours?" (3) "What are other plausible explanations for this symptom?" Or (4) "What are the reasonable steps you can take to deal with this?" It can be helpful to look at the socratic questions throughout this book to help guide you in this process.

(2) Try not to make your loved one feel guilty, punish them or assume they aren't trying to change their health anxiety.

If your loved one is reading this book, they are likely trying to change. Improving health anxiety isn't easy and takes time. Getting angry at them will only slow their progress. It further complicates the process, as this can lead them to experience other unpleasant emotions on top of anxiety. People with anxiety can't be guilted into not having anxiety. Try to have compassion and understanding, especially if they are putting in the work to get better. We all have our own struggles. It can sometimes be helpful to remind yourself of the struggles you have that they (hopefully) try to be compassionate and understanding about. We are all a work in progress!

All that said, it is worth noting that you are human too and it is understandable that you will lose patience at times. When you notice this happening, try to seek your own support and take space when you need it. Lastly, don't blame yourself either. Your loved ones' health anxiety progress is not in your control. Focus on what you can control, such as taking those steps to provide support and encourage them to work on it.

(3) Don't tease or make fun of your loved one for their health anxiety

Try not to mock them or call them "crazy," "neurotic" or assume they are faking an illness for attention. There is a long history of people with health anxiety being mocked and misunderstood. Health anxiety has often been made fun of in mainstream culture ("Oh, he is *such* a hypochondriac."). In fact, the term "hypochondriasis" was removed from the diagnostic statistical manual of mental disorders for this reason: it portrayed the experience of health anxiety as something bizarre and comical and, consequently, stigmatized people who were already feeling alone and misunderstood. In reality, many people struggle with health anxiety to varying degrees and it is something to be taken seriously, similar to depression, PTSD or any other mental health struggle. Instead of contributing to the stigma and shame they have likely already experienced, it can be helpful to help them feel safe, understood and supported.

In addition, the expressed concerns and behaviors of those with health anxiety is sometimes assumed to be a method for seeking attention (similar to those with Fictitious Disorder, formerly known as Munchaesen

Syndrome). However, this is false. People with health anxiety want more than anything to *not* have an illness. Although some of their actions might mirror those with Fictitious Disorder/Munchaesen Syndrome (e.g. frequent doctor visits, repeatedly talking about symptoms), the ultimate goal of those with health anxiety is not to receive attention but simply to make sure they are safe and okay. It is important that you understand these key distinctions so you don't make inaccurate assumptions about their thoughts and behaviors. Again, a valuable way to support someone with health anxiety is to better understand them and their experiences.

Helpful Responses or "Dos"

(1) Try to understand more about why your loved one is worried about their health and how the anxiety feeds itself.

There is a lot more going on behind the scenes with health anxiety than we realize. It can be helpful to try to understand more about this. Specifically, your loved one has unique core fears, triggers, thoughts, beliefs and unhelpful coping mechanisms. This all contributes to a vicious cycle. Understanding more about this can help you have more compassion, empathy as well as help you know how to approach the situation more productively. Therefore, it might be helpful to read CBT books (like this one) about health anxiety that go into detail about this. If your health-anxious loved one is in therapy, it can also be helpful to join them in a therapy session so you can learn more about why they think, feel and behave the way they do when it comes to health-related situations.

(2) When relevant, provide praise and encouragement for any progress your loved one makes with their health anxiety, even in small ways or minor, everyday situations.

Getting better isn't easy. It takes a lot of determination, courage and discipline to make lasting change with health anxiety. This typically involves making small changes each day in their thoughts, beliefs and behaviors. Given that it is difficult and requires persistence, it can be helpful when you notice the small "wins" or progress and encourage your loved one to continue. It can also be helpful if you remind them of their progress on the hard days when they slip back into old patterns (which will happen at times, even though they are on the path to getting better).

(3) Allow yourself to seek additional support or take breaks and engage in self-care as you support your loved one with health anxiety.

As you may know, living with health anxiety is not only exhausting for the sufferer but for loved ones as well. It can consume large chunks of time and energy. Similar to when you are dealing with any type of challenging situation, it may be helpful to get additional support through therapy, support groups or other loved ones. This will give you the space to talk about what has been difficult, giving you the emotional outlet you likely need. This may lead to less frustration, resentment and burn out, particularly on the harder days. It may also help improve your compassion and capacity to deal with the day-to-day struggle of loving someone with health anxiety.

Guide/Tips for Finding a Therapist

Finding a therapist can often feel like a challenging and overwhelming task, but there are numerous resources available to simplify the process. Online tools and directories provide a wide range of options, allowing you to tailor your search to your unique needs. Many platforms let you filter therapists based on factors such as insurance, areas of expertise, therapeutic approaches, cost, and even personal identity considerations. Additionally, professional associations and local organizations often maintain directories or offer referrals.

Below is a curated list of resources to help you navigate the journey of finding a therapist that's right for you.

Therapist Directories

These directories provide comprehensive search features to help you find therapists based on various criteria.

- **Psychology Today**: A popular directory with detailed filters for insurance, issues, therapy types, and more.
- **Good Therapy**: Focuses on ethical therapy practices and includes a robust therapist search tool.
- **Therapy Den**: An inclusive directory with filters for specific populations, such as LGBTQ+ clients.
- **BetterHelp**: Connects users to licensed therapists for online counseling services.
- **Open Path Collective**: Offers affordable in-person and online therapy options.

- **Network Therapy**: Features therapists specializing in a wide range of mental health issues.
- **Find A Therapist**: Helps you locate professionals by location or specialty.
- **Therapy Tribe**: A community-driven platform offering therapist search options.
- **Theravive**: Includes detailed profiles of licensed professionals.
- **Mental Health Match**: Matches clients with therapists based on needs and preferences.
- **Zencare**: Offers a streamlined process to find vetted therapists.
- **Inclusive Therapists**: Focuses on diverse and culturally responsive care.
- **Therapists for Black Girls**: A directory and supportive community for Black women.
- **The Black Emotional and Mental Health Collective (BEAM)**: Connects individuals to Black mental health professionals.
- **Therapy for Black Men**: A resource to support mental health care for Black men.
- **Therapy for Latinx**: A platform to find Latinx-focused therapists.
- **The Asian Mental Health Collective**: Focuses on connecting Asian clients to mental health resources.
- **Melanin & Mental Health**: Highlights therapists of color for clients of color.
- **The National Queer & Trans Therapists of Color Network**: Provides a directory of therapists for queer and trans people of color.

Find Therapists Through Associations and Organizations

Professional organizations often maintain directories or referral services to connect individuals with qualified mental health providers.

- **Anxiety and Depression Association of America (ADAA)**: Offers resources and a directory for anxiety and depression treatments.
- **Beck Institute for Cognitive Behavior Therapy**: Find CBT practitioners trained by the Beck Institute.
- **Academy of Cognitive Therapy**: Includes certified cognitive therapists.
- **American Psychological Association (APA)**: Features a psychologist locator service.

- **National Register of Health Service Psychologists**: Offers a searchable database of licensed psychologists.
- **National Alliance on Mental Illness (NAMI)**: Provides local resources and directories.
- **National Institute of Mental Health (NIMH)**: Offers a range of mental health resources.
- **The Trevor Project**: A vital resource for LGBTQ+ youth mental health support.
- **Substance Abuse and Mental Health Services Administration (SAMHSA)**: Includes a locator for treatment centers and mental health professionals.

Additional Avenues to Find Therapists

If online directories aren't sufficient, consider exploring these options:

- **Churches or Religious Organizations**: Many faith-based organizations provide or refer to mental health services.
- **Local Community Organizations:** Nonprofits and local groups often host mental health programs or provide therapist referrals.
- **Insurance Company Directory**: Most insurance providers maintain a list of in-network mental health professionals.

Final Tips

- Be patient and persistent in your search; finding the right therapist takes time.
- Reach out to multiple therapists for consultations to determine who feels like the best fit before making a commitment (many therapists offer free phone consultations). While a therapist's skill and expertise are essential, finding someone with whom you feel comfortable and understood is equally important for a successful therapeutic relationship.
- Don't hesitate to ask questions about a therapist's experience, approach, or specialties to ensure they align with your needs. Specifically for health anxiety, I would encourage you to ask whether they use CBT techniques (if the techniques in this book have been helpful for you). If they say yes, ask more about the specific techniques they use. Do they use cognitive restructuring techniques (e.g., core belief worksheets, socratic dialogue, examine the evidence

exercises)? Do they help reduce the use of avoidance and safety behaviors with experiments and exposure tasks?

Taking the first step to seek help is a courageous move—utilize these resources to make the journey smoother and more rewarding.

Navigating the Cost of Therapy

For many, the cost of therapy can feel like a significant obstacle. However, there are various options and resources available to make therapy more accessible and affordable. Below is a more detailed look at the different ways to manage the cost of mental health services.

1 Self-Pay
Paying out of pocket, or self-paying, allows for greater flexibility in choosing a therapist. While this can sometimes be expensive, some therapists offer sliding-scale fees based on income or financial circumstances. This approach is ideal for those who prefer to bypass insurance limitations or seek specialized care that may not be covered by their insurance plan.

2 Using Insurance
Many insurance plans include mental health benefits. Here are key points to consider:

- **In-Network Providers**: Insurance companies often have a list of therapists within their network, which can significantly reduce costs.
- **Out-of-Network Providers**: Some plans offer partial reimbursement for therapists outside the network. Check with your insurer for details.
- **Telehealth Services**: Many insurance plans now cover online therapy sessions. Before scheduling an appointment, confirm the therapist's acceptance of your insurance and understand your co-pay or deductible.

3 App-Based Therapy Providers
Therapy apps like **BetterHelp**, **Talkspace**, and others provide affordable alternatives to traditional therapy. These platforms typically offer:

- Lower costs than in-person sessions.
- Flexible communication options (text, video, or audio).
- Subscription models with varying levels of support.

4 Free or Low-Cost Therapy Services

There are numerous organizations and programs that offer therapy at little to no cost:

- **Mental Health America (MHA)**: Provides resources and tools to connect individuals with free or low-cost mental health care.
- **Open Path Collective**: Offers access to affordable therapy, with rates ranging from $30–$60 per session.
- **Local Non-Profit Organizations**: Many nonprofits provide free or reduced-cost therapy services. Check within your community for options.
- **University or College Counseling Centers**: Many higher education institutions offer free or low-cost therapy to students, faculty, and sometimes the local community.
- **Federally Subsidized Health Centers**: Community health centers funded by the federal government often include free or sliding-scale mental health services. Search for local centers through the Health Resources and Services Administration (HRSA) website.

5 Employee Assistance Programs (EAPs)

If you're employed, your workplace may offer an **Employee Assistance Program (EAP)** as part of your benefits package. Key features include:

- Short-term counseling services, usually ranging from 3–7 sessions.
- Support for mental health, work-life balance, and personal challenges.
- Confidential and free to employees. Contact your HR department to learn more about accessing EAP services.

6 Sliding Scale and Reduced-Fee Therapy

Some private practice therapists provide sliding-scale payment options based on your income. This is a great way to access high-quality care at a reduced cost. Many therapists list this information on their profiles in directories like Psychology Today or Therapy Den, or you can inquire directly when reaching out.

Resources for Psychiatric Medication

Understanding mental health medications can be overwhelming, but with the right resources and strategies, you can access reliable information to make informed decisions. Below is a list of tips and trusted resources to help you learn more about psychiatric medications, their uses, side effects, and management.

Tips for Finding Information About Mental Health Medications

1 Consult a Healthcare Professional

- **Primary Care Provider (PCP)**: They can often provide initial guidance or referrals to a psychiatrist.
- **Psychiatrist**: As specialists in mental health, psychiatrists are best equipped to diagnose and prescribe medications.
- **Pharmacist**: Pharmacists are an excellent resource for understanding medication side effects, interactions, and usage instructions.

2 Request a Comprehensive Review

- Ask your provider to explain the purpose, benefits, potential side effects, and alternatives for any prescribed medication.
- Inquire about interactions with other medications or supplements you may be taking.

3 Use Reliable Online Resources

- Look for information from well-regarded medical and mental health organizations rather than forums or unverified sources.

4 Understand Your Prescription

- Read the medication guide provided with your prescription. It contains detailed information about dosage, warnings, and side effects.

5 Join Support Groups or Communities

- Peer groups, whether in-person or online, can provide real-world insights into managing mental health medications.

Resources for Medication Information

1 U.S. Government and Health Organization Websites

- **MedlinePlus**: A service of the National Library of Medicine offering drug information, side effects, and interactions.
- **FDA - Mental Health Medications**: Information on FDA-approved psychiatric medications, safety updates, and recalls.

- **National Institute of Mental Health (NIMH)**: Provides resources on medication types, their uses, and general mental health information.
- **SAMHSA Medication-Assisted Treatment**: Covers medications used for substance use disorders and co-occurring mental health issues.

2 Professional Organizations

- **NAMI (National Alliance on Mental Illness)**: Offers easy-to-understand guides on common psychiatric medications and their uses.
- **Mental Health America (MHA)**: Provides information about medication options, side effects, and coping strategies.
- **American Psychiatric Association (APA)**: Resources for understanding psychiatric medications and best practices.
- **American Academy of Child & Adolescent Psychiatry (AACAP)**: Information on medications specifically for children and teens.

3 Medication and Drug Information Databases

- **Drugs.com**: Offers a comprehensive database with details about prescription and over-the-counter medications.
- **RxList**: Provides detailed information about medications, including uses, side effects, and interactions.
- **PDR (Physicians' Desk Reference) Online**: A trusted source for in-depth drug information, commonly used by healthcare professionals.

4 Mobile Apps

- **MediSafe**: A medication management app with reminders and education about your prescriptions.
- **Drugs.com Medication Guide**: Offers detailed drug information, a pill identifier, and interaction checker.

Questions to Ask Your Healthcare Provider

- What is the purpose of this medication, and how does it work?
- What are the most common side effects, and how can I manage them?
- Are there lifestyle changes I should make while taking this medication?
- How long will it take for the medication to start working?
- What should I do if I miss a dose?
- Are there alternative medications or treatments available?

Final Tips

- Be proactive in learning about your medication, but avoid self-diagnosing or altering your treatment without consulting a professional.
- Stay organized by keeping a medication log, noting dosages, schedules, and any side effects you experience.
- If affordability is a concern, explore patient assistance programs offered by pharmaceutical companies or organizations like NeedyMeds or RxAssist.

Being informed about mental health medications empowers you to advocate for yourself and engage actively in your treatment journey.

Finding Support Groups for Health Anxiety

Support groups can be a valuable resource for individuals struggling with health anxiety, offering understanding, encouragement, and practical coping strategies. Below is a list of tips and resources to help you find the right support group for your needs.

Tips for Finding Support Groups

1 Determine Your Preferences

- Decide whether you prefer in-person or online groups.
- Consider the size of the group and the level of interaction you're comfortable with.

2 Look for Groups Specific to Health Anxiety

- Seek groups that focus specifically on health anxiety or related conditions like generalized anxiety disorder (GAD) or obsessive-compulsive disorder (OCD).

3 Start Locally

- Check with local hospitals, mental health clinics, or community centers for support groups in your area.
- Ask your therapist or healthcare provider for recommendations.

4 Explore Online Options

- Online support groups offer flexibility and anonymity, making it easier to connect with others from the comfort of your home.

5 Verify the Credibility of the Group

- Look for groups moderated by professionals or backed by reputable mental health organizations.
- Avoid forums or groups that promote unverified medical advice or fear-based discussions.
- Avoid forums or groups that allow reassurance-seeking about symptoms

Resources for Finding Support Groups

1 Online Support Groups

- **International OCD ASoA Health Anxiety Support Group** Offers a weekly online support group for health anxiety, led by licensed therapists/health anxiety experts
- **Anxiety and Depression Association of America (ADAA)** Offers a list of online support groups and resources specifically for anxiety
- **No More Panic** A UK-based website with forums and resources for those experiencing health anxiety and panic disorders.
- **The Tribe – Support Groups** Offers free online groups for individuals coping with health anxiety and other mental health challenges.
- **Grouport** Offers online therapy groups for individuals coping with health anxiety and other mental health challenges.

2 Local Support Group Directories

- **NAMI (National Alliance on Mental Illness)** Provides a database of local support groups, including those for anxiety disorders, across the U.S.
- **Mental Health America (MHA)** Offers a searchable directory of mental health resources, including support groups.
- **Psychology Today** Offers a searchable directory of mental health resources, including searching for local support groups by zip code.

3 Therapy-Based Groups

- **Cognitive Behavioral Therapy (CBT), Acceptance and Commitment Therapy (ACT) and Other Groups**: Many therapists offer group CBT sessions focused on anxiety management. Check with local therapists or clinics.
- **Hospitals and Mental Health Clinics**: These institutions often host group therapy sessions or peer-led support groups.

4 **Social Media/Online Communities**

- **Facebook Groups**: Search for health anxiety-specific groups, such as "Health Anxiety Support" or "Living with Anxiety."
- **Reddit**: Subreddits like r/healthanxiety provide a space for sharing experiences and coping strategies.
- **Anxiety UK**: Offers support group information, including resources for those experiencing health anxiety.
- **Meetup**: Search for local anxiety or mental health support meetups in your area.

Note, be cautious with joining peer-led groups that aren't moderated by mental health professionals. You do not want to join online forums or groups that promote/permit activities that will only increase your health anxiety (e.g. seeking reassurance about symptoms, sharing experiences that perpetuate fear and misinformation). This could end up being counterproductive.

Additional Tips for Making the Most of a Support Group

- **Be Open and Honest**: Share your experiences to gain meaningful insights and build connections.
- **Set Boundaries**: Participate at a level that feels comfortable for you; it's okay to start by just listening.
- **Focus on Positivity**: Engage with groups that emphasize support, solutions, and encouragement rather than promote fear and dependency.

Patient Advocacy Resources

Patient advocacy services can be a valuable resource for individuals navigating the complexities of the healthcare system. Advocates provide support in understanding medical information, managing insurance issues, coordinating care, and ensuring patients' rights are respected. Below are tips and resources to help you access patient advocacy services.

Tips for Accessing Patient Advocacy Services

1 **Start with Your Healthcare Provider**

- Many hospitals and clinics have patient advocacy offices or representatives who can assist with concerns, billing issues, or care coordination.

- Ask your primary care provider or specialist if they offer advocacy support within their practice.

2 **Contact Your Insurance Company**

- Health insurance providers often have case managers or patient advocates to help you navigate coverage, claims, and appeals.

3 **Explore National and Local Advocacy Organizations**

- Numerous organizations specialize in advocating for patients with specific conditions or general healthcare needs.

4 **Hire a Private Patient Advocate**

- Independent advocates provide personalized support, from reviewing medical bills to attending appointments with you.
- Look for certified advocates to ensure professionalism and expertise.

5 **Leverage Community Resources**

- Many community-based organizations, including nonprofits, offer free or low-cost patient advocacy services.

Trusted Resources for Patient Advocacy Services

1 **Hospital and Healthcare System Advocates**

- **Patient Relations Departments**: Available at most hospitals, these teams address complaints, clarify care plans, and ensure patient rights.
- **Social Workers**: Often part of the care team, social workers can assist with advocacy, resource connections, and emotional support.
- **Case Managers**: Many healthcare facilities assign case managers to help with post-discharge planning and care coordination.

2 **National Patient Advocacy Organizations**

- **National Patient Advocate Foundation (NPAF)**: Offers resources and policy advocacy for patients navigating healthcare challenges.
- **Patient Advocate Foundation (PAF)**: Provides direct assistance with insurance disputes, medical debt, and access to care.
- **Medicare Rights Center**: Assists Medicare beneficiaries with coverage questions, appeals, and education.

3 **Condition-Specific Advocacy Groups**

- **CancerCare**: Provides advocacy and financial support for individuals affected by cancer.
- **American Diabetes Association**: Offers advocacy services and resources for people with diabetes.
- **National Alliance on Mental Illness (NAMI)**: Provides advocacy support for mental health care access and insurance issues.

4 **Independent Patient Advocacy Services**

- **Greater National Advocates**: A directory of independent patient advocates certified to assist with medical and insurance navigation.
- **The Alliance of Professional Health Advocates (APHA)**: Connects patients to trained, professional advocates in their area.
- **AdvoConnection**: A searchable database of private patient advocates across the U.S.

5 **Insurance and Government Programs**

- **State Health Insurance Assistance Programs (SHIP)**: Provides free counseling and advocacy for Medicare beneficiaries.
- **Healthcare.gov**: Offers guidance for individuals navigating insurance plans through the marketplace.
- **Medicaid Offices**: State Medicaid offices often provide advocacy or connect you with relevant resources.

6 **Community and Nonprofit Resources**

- **211.org**: A nationwide service that connects individuals to local resources, including patient advocacy.
- **Legal Aid Societies**: Many legal aid organizations offer assistance with healthcare rights and disputes.
- **Local Area Agencies on Aging (AAA)**: For seniors, AAAs provide advocacy and support for accessing healthcare and related services.

How Patient Advocates Can Help

Patient advocates provide support in areas such as:

- **Insurance Navigation**: Help with understanding benefits, filing claims, and appealing denials.

- **Care Coordination**: Assist in managing appointments, treatments, and communication between providers.
- **Medical Bill Review**: Identify errors or negotiate with providers for lower costs.
- **Rights and Education**: Ensure you understand your rights as a patient and help you make informed decisions about your care.
- **Emotional Support**: Offer guidance and reassurance during challenging medical situations.

Questions to Ask When Choosing a Patient Advocate

- Are you certified or part of a professional organization?
- What are your areas of expertise?
- What is your fee structure? (if hiring a private advocate)
- How will you communicate and keep me informed?
- Can you provide references or success stories?

Patient advocacy services empower individuals to navigate the healthcare system with confidence and ensure their voices are heard. Whether you need help understanding insurance, resolving billing disputes, or managing your care, these resources can provide essential support.

Index